THE CHALLENGES OF
LUPUS
INSIGHTS & HOPE

D1249599

HENRIETTA ALADJEM

AVERY PUBLISHING GROUP

Garden City Park • New York

The information, advice, and procedures contained in this book are based upon the research and the personal and professional experiences of the authors. They are not intended as a substitute for consulting with your physician or other health-care provider. The publisher and author are not responsible for any adverse effects or consequences resulting from the use of any of the suggestions, preparations, or procedures discussed in this book. All matters pertaining to your physical health should be supervised by a health care professional. It is a sign of wisdom, not cowardice, to seek a second or third opnion.

Cover designer: Eric Macaluso
In-house editor: Dara Stewart
Typesetter: Gary A. Rosenberg and Elaine V. McCaw
Printer: Paragon Press, Honesdale, PA

Avery Publishing Group
120 Old Broadway
Garden City Park, NY 11040
1–800–548–5757
www.averypublishing.com

Library of Congress Cataloging-in-Publication Data

Aladjem, Henrietta, 1917–
    The challenges of lupus: insights and hope / Henrietta Aladjem
       p.   cm.
    Includes index.
    ISBN 0-89529-881-3
    1. Systemic lupus erythematosus—Popular works. I. Title.
    RC924.5.L85A3828   1999
    616.7'7—dc21   98-47123
                                             CIP

Printed in the United States of America

10 9 8 7 6 5 4 3

Contents

PART FOUR—MANIFESTATIONS OF LUPUS

PART FIVE—LUPUS: ITS DIAGNOSIS AND MEDICATIONS USED TO TREAT IT

PART SIX—THE DOCTOR-PATIENT RELATIONSHIP

The Challenges of Lupus *is dedicated to Janine André Schwartz and Lisa Hamel. Each in her own way has exemplified the drive and dedication to goals that enable us to envision an optimistic future for today's patient with systemic lupus erythematosus. Janine, a physician and medical scientist at Tufts-New England Medical Center, worked tirelessly to uncover new information applicable to understanding immune mechanisms in health and disease. Lisa, motivated by her own affliction with lupus, strove to become a scientist, a field to which Janine gave special meaning. Sadly, Lisa's vision as a science student at Simmons College was not to be realized. Recalling their untimely passings evokes fond remembrances, admiration, and appreciation.*

Contributors

Chester Alper, M.D., Senior Associate in Hematology and Oncology, Department of Medicine, Children's Hospital, Boston; Professor of Pediatrics, Harvard Medical School; Associate Director, The Center for Blood Research, Inc.

T. Stephen Balch, M.D., F.A.C.P., Director, Lupus Clinic, Atlanta, Georgia; Former Chair, Education Committee, Lupus Foundation of America, Inc.

Judah A. Denburg, M.D., F.R.C.P.C., Professor, Department of Medicine, McMaster University, Toronto, Canada.

Neil F. Duane, Past President, Medical Writer's Association, New England Chapter.

Carmen G. Espinoza, M.D., Professor of Pathology, Louisiana State University Medical School.

Luis R. Espinoza, M.D., Professor and Chief, Section of Rheumatology, LSU School of Medicine, New Orleans.

Elizabeth Petri Henske, M.D., Associate Member, Fox Chase Center, Philadelphia, Pennsylvania.

Graham R.V. Hughes, M.D., F.R.C.P., Lupus Research Unit, The Payne Institute, St. Thomas' Hospital, London.

Stephen R. Kaplan, M.D., F.A.C.P., Department of Medicine, Millard Fillmore Hospital, Buffalo, New York.

Robert S. Katz, M.D., Associate Professor of Medicine, Rush Medical School in Chicago; Chair of the LFA Education Committee.

Stephen I. Katz, M.D., Ph.D., Director of the National Institute of Arthritis and Musculoskeletal and Skin Diseases, National Institutes of Health, Bethesda, Maryland.

Shah Khoshbin, M.D., Department of Neurology, Brigham and Women's Hospital; Professor, Harvard Medical School.

Steven J. Kingsbury, M.D., Ph.D., Associate Professor in Psychiatry, University of Texas, Southwestern Medical School.

Robert G. Lahita, M.D., Ph.D., Associate Professor of Medicine, Columbia University; Chief of Rheumatology and Connective Tissue Diseases, Saint Luke's Roosevelt Hospital.

Michael D. Lockshin, M.D., F.A.C.P., Director, Barbara Volcker Center for Women and Rheumatic Disease; Professor of Medicine, Hospital for Special Surgery, Cornell University Medical School, New York.

Michelle Petri, M.D., M.P.H., Associate Professor of Medicine, Johns Hopkins University School of Medicine, Baltimore, Maryland.

Malcolm P. Rogers, M.D., Associate Professor of Psychiatry, Harvard Medical School.

Naomi Rothfield, M.D., Professor of Medicine and Chief, Division of Rheumatic Diseases, the University of Connecticut Health Center.

Peter H. Schur, M.D., Professor of Medicine, Harvard Medical School; Senior Physician at Brigham and Women's Hospital; Director, Lupus Clinic and Research.

Robert S. Schwartz, M.D., Associate Editor, New England Medical Journal.

Howard Steven Shapiro, M.D., Assistant Clinical Professor, University of Southern California School of Medicine, Department of Psychiatry and Human Behavior.

Robert B. Silver, Ph.D., Underwater Research Laboratory, Woods Hole, Massachusetts.

Daniel J. Wallace, M.D., F.A.C.P., Clinical Professor of Medicine, UCLA School of Medicine.

Robert B. Zurier, M.D., Professor of Medicine, Director, Division of Rheumatology, University of Massachusetts Memorial Health Care System.

All submitted articles in this book have been published with the kind permission of their authors.

Acknowledgments

I want to thank all the physicians who have written chapters for this book. Their contributions have shed light on this still mysterious and little understood disease. Their names are too many to list here; however, they appear in the list of contributors on the preceding page. I consider all these physicians to be my mentors, my friends, and the friends of every lupus patient.

I also want to thank the patients who have allowed me to print their personal letters in this book. Written from the heart, these letters display the core of what it is to have a chronic disease that is potentially fatal. Their writings are a great help to the members of the lupus community who now feel less isolated and alone.

I am grateful to John Lauerman who read the manuscript carefully and tamed the unruly English grammatical sentence structure, as I am still self-taught in the English language and thus lost in its maze of arbitrary and uncomfortable rules. After fifty years in this country, I sometimes still translate my thoughts from Bulgarian or French to English. John is a master of the English language.

I also want to thank Nancye Connor who has typed my manuscripts for the past twenty-two years. Her skills and devotion show in every page she produces. Nancye is a professional who works with the heart of a volunteer. I also want to thank Sam Nosratian who has been my "Man Friday" for quite a few years. I met Sam when he was a very small boy racing on a tricycle. It was love at first sight. Sam is now seventeen. He types for me, goes to the post office, buys office supplies, and does the photostatting and everything else when I need his help.

And last but not least, I must express my gratitude to my family for believing in me and my work. Without their love and moral support and encouragement, even a determined person like me could falter. I am a very fortunate person to be able to do what I like best—writing, researching, and helping to empower the lupus patient through education and public awareness.

Foreword

Systemic lupus erythematosus (also known as lupus or SLE) is in a category of diseases known as "autoimmune" diseases, in which, through some quirk of nature, the body begins to see some of its own tissues as foreign and launches an immune attack against those tissues. To the physician and the researcher, lupus is a medical puzzle—baffling, challenging, frustrating. To the individual who suffers from lupus, the disease is all that and more. First, it is a series of symptoms that must be successfully diagnosed—often a difficult task in its own right! Finally, it is an uninvited life companion that must be accepted in some ways, overcome in other ways, understood and managed minute by minute and day by day.

Henrietta Aladjem speaks to both the medical professional and the patient. As a woman with lupus, she is an example to all those who must live with chronic illness, and who seek to rise above it. As a serious student of the disease, she speaks plainly and humanely to medical professionals who treat and investigate this disease, giving it a human face and an understandable vocabulary.

She knows that patients themselves have a critical role in managing their own chronic diseases like lupus. Studies have shown repeatedly that those patients who have self-efficacy—who understand and take control of their diseases—are able to manage their diseases better. Information is power—and information for patients is empowering.

And it is because information is power that I am pleased by the program of research into lupus and other autoimmune diseases that is carried out by my department. America is investing wisely in its support for research at our National Institutes of Health (NIH) and other Health and Human Services agencies. In addition to basic research and clinical trials, NIH supports a registry for patients with lupus as well as a repository for genetic material from patients and their families to enable the identification of the genes involved in lupus. I am confident that it will be through the contributions of studies in each of these areas that we will finally come to understand the total puzzle of diseases like lupus.

And as we learn, we must share our new knowledge in every way possible. Research is of very limited value if the results never get to patients and their doctors. We are committed to disseminating results widely and to targeting particularly vulnerable communties—as we have done, for example, in targeting African-American women, who have an increased susceptibility to lupus.

We will continue to learn more about lupus. We will continue to share that vital information with all those who need it. And we will continue to draw strength and understanding from those, like Ms. Aladjem, who speak to us from their experience, their trials, and their triumphs.

—Donna E. Shalala
U.S. Secretary of Health and Human Services

Preface

In 1972, I wrote *The Sun Is My Enemy,* a detailed account of my own lupus story, so that others might read it and benefit from my experiences. All the doctors I had consulted had told me that systemic lupus erythematosus was a rare disease of obscure origin and of short duration that was fatal. If the patient didn't die within three or four years, the physician questioned the diagnosis.

I became the victim of my own environment: My skin needed protection from the heat, cold, wind, ultraviolet light, anything that touched it. The drugs I took, instead of helping, caused more problems, which were never interpreted correctly. These reactions should have been received as a warning signal from nature, not just for some drugs, but for all. I was susceptible to infections, and I had to cope with an overactive immune system that was playing havoc with my health. Instead of producing antibodies against foreign invaders, such as bacteria or viruses, I was producing antibodies against my body's own constituents, my own tissue.

For years and years, I have been affected by an illness with an unpronouncable name, of unknown causes, and with symptoms that were difficult to explain. But I was also fortunate to have had a good physician and a supportive family. I didn't have to go to work every day to earn a living; I could stay at home to take care of myself and my children. And I am lucky to have been in complete remission for over twenty years. By a complete remission, I mean I have not needed to take any medications and my medical tests have shown no signs of illness.

Over the years, I have developed a deep sense of my own experiences with lupus, and I have also absorbed the sufferings of the patients I came to know. I have read their sad letters, and I have heard their crying voices in person and over the telephone. Some of their stories have appeared in *Understanding Lupus,* another book that I wrote on the subject.

Many of the lupus patients express their discontent with the medical profession. They tell me that there is a need for a doctor who can listen to them and explain things in a comprehensible language. They say that one needs a physician who can practice the art of medicine as well as the science of medicine, and we also need a physician who will take care of us in the intensive care unit as well as help us with chronic illness. Disease deals with lab tests and studies under the microscopes, while illness is how the patient survives on a daily basis when one is burdened with psychosocial problems, with economic difficulties, and with the physical discomfort created by the disease.

Perhaps I should describe a real-life situation I had to face at a lupus seminar in Boston. I met a patient there whom I don't believe I shall ever forget. Her name was Mrs. White. Mrs. White's face, neck, arms, skull, and lips were covered with oozing boils and sores. She looked like a reincarnation of the biblical figure Job, who was forced to suffer several calamities, or someone who had walked out of a nightmare. I shivered with pain just looking at her. Mrs. White had lupus vulgaris, also known as tuberculosis of the skin, a condition rarely seen today.

I asked Mrs. White what she was doing for her sores. She said she sees a doctor at a major hospital in Boston. He gave her a prescription for a salve to apply all over her body after she soaked for a half hour in a tub full of hot water. However, Mrs. White lived in an apartment that had neither a bathtub nor hot water. I asked her if her doctor knew about her situation. Mrs. White said he gave her the prescription with a sheet of instructions before he whisked her out of the office to attend to another patient in the examining room.

"He is always overbooked," she said. "His waiting room is crowded with patients." She said she waited for months for an appointment, only to be seen by him for about ten minutes, and, she said, he spent half of that time writing in a notebook. Mrs. White said, "I feel tongue-tied when I am with him, and when I leave his office, I cry. I cry with dry eyes, for I can't make tears in my eyes or saliva in my mouth due to my illness." She shook her head sadly before there was a wisp of a smile over her dry lips. I felt guilty when my own eyes began filling up with moisture.

I've read in a book by the late Dr. Rene Dubós, editor of the *Journal of Experimental Medicine,* that the hope in the future lies in the physician's willingness to listen to the patient, and the patient's courage to reject medical science without humanity. This brings to mind something Dr. Richard Krause, Senior Science Advisor at Fogarty International Center at the National Institutes of Health in Bethesda, Maryland, once said: "Along with the therapeutic marvels of the last few decades, the physician must also add to his black bag a portion of *therapeuein,* the Greek word from which the word therapy was derived, meaning a companion in attendance—a friend."

In writing this manuscript, I have compiled papers written by medical scientists, clinicians, and psychiatrists; stories written by lupus patients; and some of my own experiences with lupus that have led to my remission. The book is broken up into six parts. Part One is an introduction to the book and provides you with an overview of lupus. Part Two details my personal experiences with lupus, as well as the experiences of others with the disease. Part Three discusses the way lupus affects different groups of people at different stages of life; for example, men, children, pregnant women, and the elderly. Part Four explains the different manifestations of lupus—the way lupus affects the skin, the kidneys, the lungs, the central nervous system, etc. Part Five discusses the several medications that lupus patients so often must take. Part Six examines the importance of the doctor-patient relationship. The chapters written by physicians on understanding lupus are up-to-date and are written in a language that we can all understand. Some of the *dramatis per-*

sonae have fictitious names, while others, who remain closer to the flow of events, appropriately appear as themselves. In recreating dialogue, I have quoted from memory, and I trust I have not misrepresented their opinion or intentions. I invite you to read this book with an open mind and heart and draw inspiration from the saga of the lupus patient who chooses to live, no matter how bumpy the road.

In Sofia, Bulgaria, where I grew up, we thought of a hospital as a house of God, a doctor was both a teacher and a healer, a nurse was a sister of mercy, and a patient was referred to as a patient—never as a client. The home and the family were your security, and if you needed hospitalization, you were taken care of. I have not been back home for over fifty years, and I can't be sure anymore whether I am imagining these statements . . . or whether they are reflections of a past that does not exist anymore.

PART ONE

Lupus:
An Introduction

1

Lupus:
An Overview

by Michael D. Lockshin, M.D., F.A.C.P.

Lupus? Systemic lupus erythematosus? When you first heard those words, you probably thought, "What a funny name!" Chances are, the words meant very little to you. The name told nothing of pain or disfigurement, nor of a lifetime of thinking about health. The words could not have suggested, the first time you heard them, personal struggles against ignorance, or battles to stay confident when employers, insurers, friends, and family over- or under-interpret the portent of the diagnosis. What do the strange words mean?

WHAT IS LUPUS?

Lupus is an autoimmune disease in which one's immune system sees its own body as a foreign invader and attacks it. It can affect several different systems of the body. Currently, the illness has no known cause or cure. Lupus can be serious or trivial; disfiguring or unnoticeable; painful or painless; life-threatening or of little consequence. It can be simple to diagnose or devilishly difficult. It can be easy to treat or exceedingly hard. There are many things that lupus is *not*. Lupus is *not* contagious. It is *not* (and has nothing to do with) a venereal disease. It is *not* (and has nothing to do with) AIDS. It is *not* (and has nothing to do with) cancer. For some questions about lupus, there is no clear yes or no answer. For instance, "Can lupus be inherited?" The answer: To some degree, it appears that it can be. It's a complicated question. Another: Can patients live normal lives? The answer: Most do.

Lupus is the Latin word for *wolf.* For over one thousand years, this animal's name has described a rash on the face. It is a bit of a mystery why the name is used. Some people think that it describes what someone looks like after being attacked by a wolf. (I have never seen someone bitten by a wolf, but I have seen dog bites, and they don't look anything like a lupus rash.) Others think the rash makes a person look like a wolf. (That definitely is not true.) A third guess is that the way in which some deep infections of facial skin (not what we know today as lupus) destroy tissue somehow resembles the destruction that wolves can do. The word *erythematosus* means red, which lupus rashes are. Whatever the reason for the name, lupus rashes are not nearly as ugly as the name implies. In most patients, the rash heals leaving no trace. Many patients get no rash at all.

Lupus is not a new disease. Doctors have diagnosed lupus as we now know it—rash, arthritis, kidney inflammation, primarily in young women—since at least the mid-nineteenth century, when modern medicine began. There is serious speculation by medical historians that Queen Anne of England had lupus (she had recurrent arthritis and rash), and less believable speculation that Wolfgang Amadeus Mozart and Jack London had it as well. The author Flannery O'Connor suffered from lupus. Many literary critics think her experience with the disease markedly influenced her stories.

WHO GETS LUPUS?

Lupus can affect anyone. Lupus occurs in babies and octogenarians, in women and men, in blacks and whites, and in rich and poor people. A more informative answer is: Most lupus patients are young women, with about 90 percent between the ages of fifteen and forty-five. No one knows the reason why. There is much research ongoing to find out why this is so, and many good guesses. The best guess is that the disease has something to do with female hormones. Women differ from men in ways other than hormones, so other explanations are also possible. Men who get lupus are normal men. Except for a rare group of men who are born with an extra female chromosome and are unusually susceptible to lupus, men with lupus father children and are in other respects sexually normal. Mice can be bred to develop lupus. In several breeds, females develop lupus, but in one breed males do, so susceptibility to lupus might have something to do with a gene that is on the sex chromosome but is unrelated to gender or hormones. Researchers have looked, but so far no one seriously thinks that the cause of lupus is found in hair dyes or cosmetics or other items that are mostly used by women.

Systemic lupus erythematosus occurs everywhere in the world. In the United States, England, and the Caribbean, black women get the disease three times more often than do white women. Asians, brown-skinned people, and Native Americans get lupus about twice as often as whites. There is no good explanation for these occurrences. It may have something to do with heredity. Some researchers think lupus is rare in central Africa, a very curious point that suggests that environment has something to do with the development of the disease. Researchers have looked at what people eat but have not found any good clues—with one exception. Several years ago monkeys fed a certain type of alfalfa developed lupus symptoms. A fungus that contaminated the alfalfa was thought to be the cause, but was never definitely proven.

Dogs, mice, and monkeys get lupus—but pets do not transmit the disease to their owners, nor do owners with lupus give the disease to their pets, as the disease is not transmissible. Some medicines, particularly those used to treat high blood pressure and abnormal heart rhythms in humans, can (rarely) cause a disease that looks like lupus. Because the disease goes away when the medicine is stopped, doctors are very certain that the drug alone causes the lupus symptoms. Researchers have looked in lupus patients for possible exposure to naturally occurring chemicals that might be similar to the blood pressure and heart drugs that cause lupus symptoms, but have found none.

HOW DOES LUPUS AFFECT THE BODY?

Lupus is a chronic disease, which means that it is an ongoing, long-lasting illness. Chronic diseases are the kind that you have to keep checking on and control with medications. Lupus tends to come and go in spells called flares (when the illness is active) and remissions (when it disappears). Medicines keep the flares under control.

Lupus is a *systemic* disease (hence the first word of the full name), meaning that it can affect several or all parts of the body. The opposite of systemic disease is *organ-specific,* affecting only one body organ—an overactive thyroid gland, for instance. Another type of lupus, called *discoid* lupus, affects only the skin. The word discoid refers to the appearance of the rash when it starts: round circles, resembling disks. People with discoid lupus almost never develop the systemic form of the disease.

For most lupus patients, the illness affects the skin, blood, and joints, and for about half, the kidneys, too. In a smaller proportion of patients, lupus affects the brain or the lining of the heart and lungs. Lupus patients get rashes, anemia, arthritis (joint inflammation), nephritis (kidney inflammation), and sometimes brain inflammation. Most patients get only a few of these symptoms. Lupus patients have abnormal antibodies in their bloodstreams. The antibodies cause inflammation wherever they land, which can be anywhere. This is why so many different types of symptoms occur. Lupus patients also fatigue easily, as tests of their physical stamina show. The severity of lupus varies considerably. In some patients and in some organs it is barely noticeable. In other patients and other organs it is severe.

The symptoms that lupus causes depend on which parts of the body are affected. The complaint that most often brings a patient to the doctor is pain. The pain is usually felt in the joints, but sometimes it is in the muscles, or there are general aches throughout the body. Skin rash, fever, abnormal blood count, and abnormal urine tests (on a routine exam) are also frequent. The rash, when it occurs, appears on the face, especially on the cheeks and bridge of the nose and on the upper arms. The hair often thins. An individual patient may have a mild rash but bad kidney disease, or the opposite, or neither, or both.

Because the disease is variable, a doctor has to examine the whole body and do a lot of blood tests to diagnose lupus. When treating a diagnosed lupus patient, a doctor has to determine whether every new symptom is due to lupus or to something else. For instance, lupus-like symptoms may be due to flu, high blood pressure, a drug the patient is taking, or other causes.

HOW IS LUPUS DIAGNOSED?

A diagnosis of lupus is based on a patient's symptoms. Blood tests confirm—they do not make—the diagnosis. Sometimes healthy people, for one reason or another, have abnormal blood tests. When that happens, an experienced doctor should examine that person closely to be certain that the person is really okay. Patients with positive blood tests and no symptoms do not have lupus and do not need treatment. A curiosity is that about 10 percent of lupus patients have a *false positive* test for syphilis. They do not have syphilis, but their blood reacts as if they did. The false positive test often is first noted years before there are any symptoms. Many people with false positive tests never develop lupus at all. If a false positive test is found, it is reasonable to do other tests (especially to be certain that the test really is falsely positive).

Doctors use a lupus patient's abnormal antibodies to test for the disease. The antibodies bind to the nucleus of cells (so they are called *anti*nuclear *a*ntibodies or ANA). ANA tests are used to screen for lupus when the disease is suspected, because someone who has a negative ANA test almost never has lupus. A positive ANA test means that a diagnosis of lupus may be possible, but positive ANA tests are very common. In fact, most people who test positive for ANA do not have lupus. To diagnose lupus in a patient with a positive ANA test, doctors look for other antibodies that only lupus patients have: antibodies to DNA (anti-*DNA* antibodies) or to a protein that attaches to DNA (anti-Sm [standing for the name *Smith*] antibody). Almost every lupus patient has *both* a positive ANA test *and* a positive test for antibody to either DNA or Sm.

Other blood and urine tests tell a doctor how a patient is doing. Since there are almost no symptoms in early lupus kidney disease, and since urine and blood tests do not tell the doctor all that he or she needs to know about the kidneys, doctors sometimes do a kidney biopsy to decide whether to treat for mild or for severe kidney disease. It is usual for doctors to keep checking blood and urine tests, even in patients who are well, to identify change as early as possible.

WHAT TRIGGERS LUPUS FLARES?

If you do not now have lupus, no matter what your parent or spouse or friend tells you, changing your lifestyle won't prevent lupus from developing nor cause it to come. Doctors do not know what causes lupus to appear, even in patients with early symptoms. On the other hand, if you do have lupus, there are certain triggers that can cause a flare of symptoms. Intense sun exposure can be one such trigger. Sensitivity to the sun occurs in about one of every three lupus patients. It varies in severity. For most sun-sensitive patients, it takes a lot of sun exposure—a day at the beach, a mid-summer afternoon on the tennis court—to cause a flare. A few people are very sun-sensitive and have to protect themselves from even a small amount of sun exposure. Using sun-blockers, staying off the tennis courts except in the early morning or late afternoon, wearing long sleeves and broad-brimmed hats on summer outings, choosing the woods instead of the beach for summer vacations, and wearing every bit of protective gear (including a ski mask) on ski vacations are all important ways of protecting oneself from sun exposure—common sense will tell you what the rules for sun-sensitive patients must be. Infections can also trigger flares, as can exhaustion and emotional stress. Lupus patients must take care to protect themselves and treat any signs of infection or illness as soon as possible.

CAN LUPUS PATIENTS LIVE NORMAL LIVES?

I brought up the question "Can lupus patients live normal lives" earlier in this article. Much of this book discusses exactly that question. Most patients, in fact, do live normal lives. Patients with lupus marry, have babies, have jobs, play sports, and do all sorts of normal things. Most live long lives. I can't say all do. That is why we still do research and why we are still looking for a cure.

CAN LUPUS BE INHERITED?

One of the hottest areas of today's lupus research is genetics. It appears that lupus is not inherited as simply as blue eyes or brown hair are, but a tendency to develop the disease is. Once one family member has been diagnosed, the risk that a second member of a family will develop lupus is very low, probably less than one percent, so there is no reason for any lupus patient to panic that her or his siblings or children or parents will also fall ill. For researchers, this genetic clue is very important. If we can find why a person has a tendency to develop lupus, we can find out how to block that susceptibility and prevent or cure the disease.

HOW DO SUPPLEMENTAL HORMONES AFFECT LUPUS?

Nobody is quite sure whether taking hormones is good or bad for lupus patients. Some doctors tell women with lupus never to take birth control pills or, after menopause, female hormones, for fear the disease will get worse. Some doctors want to treat female lupus patients with male hormones and vice versa, because some female mice with lupus get better when they are treated in that way. Other doctors think that taking female hormones does women no harm. The answers to the question of the effects of hormones in lupus patients are not yet known. Studies currently being done should, within a few years, give a clearer answer about the safety of hormones in lupus patients. It is known, however, that women who have an antibody called the antiphospholipid antibody, or lupus anticoagulant, should not take hormones because it causes them to form blood clots inside their bodies. It is easy to test for these antibodies.

HOW IS LUPUS CONTROLLED?

Some day, doctors will be able to talk about cures for lupus, but not yet. Today doctors talk about controlling the disease, keeping it in remission, and preventing flares. There are many weapons in the doctor's arsenal. The first weapon is knowledge. You must know the disease well in order to assess how severe a specific patient's illness is and thus what treatment will be best. Many people need no treatment at all. If the patient does need treatment, tailor that treatment to her specific needs. The treatment might be anti-inflammatory drugs (aspirin, ibuprofen, and the *non-steroidal anti-inflammatory drugs*, or NSAIDs), or a type of drug used to treat malaria found, coincidentally, to be effective in preventing lupus flares—the antimalarial hydroxychloroquine. In more severe cases, cortisone-type drugs (steroids) and immunosuppressives (cyclophosphamide, azathioprine, and methotrexate) may be needed. Beyond these, there are many new types of drugs being tested. Some of these will prove to be very effective. The future is bright.

Almost harder than health for the patient to deal with is the constant struggle against ignorance. People have been known to shun a patient because of her appearance or because they think she is contagious. It is hard for a patient to stay confident when employers, insurers, friends, and family are overly protective or insensitive. Some people, trying to help, won't let a healthy patient do his or her job. Some insurers refuse to cover even very well patients, adding to the patient's pain. Lupus patients often look well when they are ill. Sometimes friends or family members do not believe they are truly ill. Patients are called lazy when they desperately need to rest. Spouses, bosses, parents of teenagers, take heed— Pampering a lupus patient who says she is tired is okay! It is something that you should do. You will be thanked when she again feels well.

This book, like all of Mrs. Aladjem's books, has much to say on each of these topics. It talks to patients and to their families—and to doctors as well. Read on, and learn.

2

An Overview of Lupus and the Central Nervous System

by Malcolm P. Rogers, M.D.

It has been known for more than 100 years that people with the systemic form of lupus show signs of disease activity in the brain and spinal cord, otherwise known as the central nervous system (CNS). Seizures and psychosis, in fact, are the two main manifestations of CNS involvement that have been incorporated as part of the American Rheumatologic Association's criteria for making the diagnosis. This does not mean that all or even most patients have these manifestations; CNS abnormalities are simply some of the possible signs and symptoms upon which the diagnosis is established. There are several ways in which central nervous system involvement in lupus can manifest itself.

SEIZURES

Seizures may come in different forms. Generalized seizures—called "grand mal" or tonic-clonic seizures—are characterized by loss of consciousness, total body shaking and intermittent stiffening, incontinence, and post-ictal (after seizure) lethargy. Other seizures may be more subtle. In partial-complex seizures—or temporal lobe seizures—there may be odd smells or other sensations, perceptual distortions, altered emotional states, or staring, all without a loss of consciousness. Other partial seizures might be limited to movement or numbness in part of one arm or leg.

Grand mal seizures are dramatic and invariably lead to serious medical and neurological evaluation, especially if they are occurring for the first time in adulthood. Partial-complex seizures, on the other hand, may be misdiagnosed or simply unrecognized for long periods. The location and degree of abnormal electrical discharge from nerve cells in the brain, which is the origin of a seizure, is best diagnosed by electroencephalography (EEG), often referred to as a brain-wave test. Generally, after the onset of new seizures, a computer tomography (CT) scan or magnetic resonance imaging (MRI) of the brain is ordered to exclude other possible causes, such as tumors or abscesses. Whatever the cause, anticonvulsant medications like Dilantin, Tegretol, and Depakote are normally used for treatment.

PSYCHOSIS

The most serious psychiatric complication of lupus is psychosis. It is characterized by symptoms such as delusions, hallucinations, and a failure of "reality testing." By this, I mean a patient's failure to properly differentiate external reality from internal fantasy and perception. Delusions are characterized by fixed and clearly false beliefs, such as the belief that Martians are controlling your thoughts. Often, psychosis is associated with tremendous fear and agitation, because of imagined beliefs that one is in acute danger.

One patient named Susan began to hear voices threatening her and her children. She was convinced that the voices were coming from outside and several times went out into the woods behind her house in search of the source. Neither her husband nor her friends heard these voices, which only added to her distress. She became increasingly frantic and agitated and would sometimes yell back in response to the voices. She was eventually persuaded to come to the hospital, where an MRI scan revealed evidence of CNS involvement. She was treated with antipsychotic medications, along with increased doses of steroids. The voices and agitation quickly subsided, and she was discharged to go home only a few days later.

It is estimated that approximately 15–20 percent of patients will have a history of seizures, and a somewhat smaller percentage will have a history of psychosis during the course of their illness. Psychotic states such as Susan's episode described above are often very frightening to patients and to their family members. They generally resolve fully, as happened in her case, with treatment of the underlying lupus and appropriate anti-anxiety and antipsychotic medications, such as Ativan or Haldol.

DEPRESSION

Depression is another common disorder that occurs in people with lupus. It is important to differentiate between depression as a symptom of lupus and depression as only one symptom of a whole syndrome, characterized by a persistent sadness, hopelessness, appetite and sleep changes, guilt, social withdrawal, difficulty concentrating, difficulty making simple everyday decisions, and sometimes suicidal wishes and plans.

Marlene was diagnosed with lupus about one year ago. Partly as a result of her illness, she had broken up with a man she had been living with for close to ten years. She felt useless and hopeless about her future. She lost interest in reading and her usual curiosity about life disappeared. Nothing seemed interesting or worthwhile. She would sometimes just sit for hours unable to initiate any activities. She just wanted to be left alone. Her parents became increasingly concerned and brought her to a rheumatologist, who, in turn, promptly referred her to a psychiatrist. She immediately started taking Paxil, an antidepressant medication, and within about three weeks she began to feel more like her old self.

These kinds of depressive syndromes tend to be self-perpetuating states, unresponsive to happy events, and presumably related to underlying changes in brain neurotransmitter chemistry. There is good evidence that depression can be a direct manifestation of lupus' effects on the CNS, although in Marlene's case there was no other evidence for CNS involvement. Whatever triggers it, serious depression should be treated with antidepressant medication and/or psychotherapy (in most cases). The good news is that depression is quite responsive to the available treatment. The most commonly used antidepressant medications are the serotonin-specific reuptake inhibitors (SSRI's), such as Prozac, Paxil, Zoloft, and Luvox. There are a range of other available antidepressants. The choices are generally made on the basis of side effects of each of the medications, because they are all roughly equal in their effectiveness against depression.

COGNITIVE PROBLEMS

Cognitive problems are also common in lupus patients. In fact, most clinicians think they are probably the most common manifestation of CNS involvement. Estimates of the prevalence vary according to different populations studies and the different neuropsychological test batteries used to study them. However, many studies have shown that more than half of patients will experience cognitive difficulties—such as memory disturbance, concentration problems, word-find problems, and so forth—during the course of their illnesses.

Jane, a 42-year-old woman who was diagnosed with lupus about ten years ago, began to have difficulty remembering where she had parked her car. She also found herself making some unusual and serious errors in her job as an accountant. She tended to forget conversations with colleagues at work. These incidents were embarrassing and very upsetting to her. She wondered if she was getting Alzheimer's disease like her elderly mother. She discussed these concerns with her rheumatologist, and was referred to a psychiatrist. The psychiatrist felt that these cognitive difficulties were significant and that she had been feeling emotionally distressed only after the cognitive difficulties caused problems. Jane underwent some special memory and other cognitive testing, which confirmed that her performance had declined in several areas, particularly her short-term memory.

We see these kinds of cognitive problems in patients who do not have any awareness of their difficulties or any other current or past symptoms of CNS lupus. Whether these should be treated with high doses of prednisone or Cytoxan is controversial and depends on an assessment of the overall clinical picture and the severity of the cognitive difficulties.

OTHER EFFECTS OF CNS INVOLVEMENT

Other relatively common examples of CNS lupus involvement are unusually severe or prolonged headaches, visual disturbances, and abnormal body movements. Less commonly, lupus disturbance of the spinal cord, referred to as transverse myelitis, may cause weakness, paralysis, loss of sensation, and loss of bladder and bowel function (incontinence). Generally, clear evidence of acute and serious CNS involvement is treated with high doses of glucocorticosteroids, such as prednisone or Solumedrol. While prednisone is an important therapy in controlling this and other aspects of lupus, it can also cause some mental side effects, including insomnia, mood changes, and even psychosis when taken in high doses.

Some individuals may experience small strokes, often related to or triggered by antiphospholipid antibodies. These strokes may involve changes in speech, cognition, or motor function. Recognition of this condition is very important because anticoagulant therapy with either aspirin or Coumadin can be very helpful. In most patients, the mechanism of neuropsychiatric or CNS lupus seems to involve a more subtle and diffuse disruption in small blood vessels in the brain that allows antibodies to interact harmfully with brain tissue.

THE PSYCHOLOGICAL EFFECTS OF HAVING LUPUS

Quite apart from the issue of direct CNS involvement, there are, of course, multiple psychological issues that produce intense reactions in patients with lupus. First, although treatment has improved dramatically, lupus remains a potentially life-threatening disorder. It may also affect the appearance of patients, either directly by producing rashes, or by virtue of some of the treatments, such as prednisone. By the same token, it sometimes can produce major changes in energy and function without obvious changes in appearance. This often leads to the difficulties patients experience when they appear well, but actually feel sick. Lupus follows its own mysterious course with flare-ups and remissions that are sometimes related to stress, but sometimes seem to come out of the blue. The very uncertainty of this illness makes it difficult for people to manage their lives and plan ahead. Finally, since this is a disease primarily of women, often in the child-bearing years, there are important issues related to developing relationships, marriages, pregnancies, and careers. So there are many psychological issues which impact lupus patients and their families, producing fear, anxiety, and sleeplessness, and complicating social and sexual functioning.

Diseases that can affect the brain, and therefore the patient's mind and sense of themselves, are inherently frightening. The integrity of our brains, which obviously provide the basis for consciousness, mental function, and our unique personalities, is of utmost importance to us all. Jane's biggest fear was that she was "losing her mind." Most patients want very much to sort out whether they are reacting psychologically to a disease, or the disease, by affecting the brain directly, is causing a change in their behavior and ability to cope.

Doctors' abilities to diagnose neuropsychiatric lupus from the kinds of problems presented by Jane, Susan, and Marlene are imperfect, which is often frustrating for them and for their patients. Neuropsychological testing is probably the most sensitive type of testing, although it is an indirect means of visualizing brain activity. Such testing consists of a series of paper-and-pencil tests of memory, spatial orientation, language, and other cognitive functions, administered by a neuropsychologist. Various brain examination techniques, such as examination of cerebrospinal fluid (CSF) by lumbar puncture, EEG, MRI, or CT scans of the head are important in determining brain activity. Doctors are also trying to develop other useful diagnostic tests, such as single photon emission computer tomography (SPECT) scans or special antibody tests. These are promising but not yet fully proven diagnostic tools.

Patients with lupus may interact with psychiatrists or other mental health professionals at various points during their illnesses. Some patients may be referred to psychiatrists early on because of vague symptoms suggestive of certain psychiatric disorders. Symptoms such as difficulty concentrating, fatigue, insomnia, loss of interest and social engagement, emotional instability, headache, and a multitude of other somatic complaints can, at times, be perceived to be psychiatric or psychosomatic disorders. Or referrals may be made later on to deal with depression, anxiety, or to help sort out CNS lupus from emotional responses to the illness. Not infrequently, there can be delays and frustration in arriving at the correct or even a certain diagnosis, which in itself may lead to emotional distress. However, a referral to a mental health provider should not be perceived as unreasonable or punitive. Psychiatrists may provide important relief for some of the aspects of lupus that cause the most suffering. I think what patients need to have emphasized is the need for emotional support during a time of diagnostic uncertainty, and throughout the course of their illness. Most clinicians believe that a combination of psychological and medical care is important for the recovery of a patient with lupus or with any other chronic disease.

3

A Message of Hope

by Stephen I. Katz, M.D., Ph.D.

This is a very exciting time to be an advocate for research on lupus—the science is really moving forward with great strides and much promise. From basic laboratory benches to patient bedsides, every day we are learning more about the causes of lupus and working toward better treatments with fewer side effects.

Two of the scientific disciplines that offer particular promise at this time are genetics and immunology. Advances in both areas will increase our understanding of lupus, as well as other autoimmune diseases. We know that genetics plays a role in lupus, and we have made a number of advances in this area, including the identification of a genetic risk factor for severe lupus kidney disease in African-Americans and the localization of a gene that predisposes people to systemic lupus erythematosus. The exciting dimension of the latter advance is that this gene appears in African-Americans, Asians, and Caucasians with lupus—it crosses multiple ethnic groups, making this a potentially significant research finding. We are committed to continuing our support of studies that will tell us more about the complex genetic basis of lupus.

We know that immunological mechanisms play a vital role in the generation and perpetuation of the events that result in lupus. The National Institute of Arthritis and Musculoskeletal and Skin Diseases (NIAMS) along with many of the other institutes at the National Institutes of Health (NIH) have made a real commitment to unraveling the mysteries of the immune system—why it attacks itself in certain circumstances and how this autoimmune response can be prevented. We also recognize that lupus and other autoimmune diseases occur much more frequently in women than in men, so the NIAMS teamed with our colleagues in the National Institute of Allergy and Infectious Diseases to encourage the submission of research proposals on gender and autoimmunity. We want to determine the basis for the increased occurrence in women.

Finally, we know that lupus is one of the many autoimmune diseases—diseases in which the body produces antibodies against itself—and we also know that progress in understanding one autoimmune disease often sheds light on others. So we continue our multipronged approach to all of the diseases within our research mandate. Those prongs include basic research (so essential to making progress against disease); animal models (that have provided vital clues to human disease—

particularly in lupus); clinical trials (like the one we are currently supporting to determine the safety of estrogen supplementation in women with lupus); and epidemiologic studies (that are necessary for us to really understand diseases like lupus in the whole population). I firmly believe that progress in all of these areas that will ultimately solve the total puzzle of autoimmune diseases like lupus.

Our ultimate goal, of course, is to help patients with lupus. We are committed to identifying the cause of lupus, improving diagnosis and treatment, and developing strategies for patients coping with this challenging disease. Improving the lives of people with lupus and similar chronic diseases is of central importance to researchers and staff of the National Institute of Arthritis and Musculoskeletal and Skin Diseases.

PART TWO

Lupus:
A *Patient's*
Perspective

4

A Patient's Perspective

by Henrietta Aladjem

In 1953, I was diagnosed with systemic lupus erythematosus—or lupus, as it is better known—a little-known and little-understood disease. I had never heard the word lupus before nor known of anyone who had anything similar to what I had. I was told that I was suffering from a rare, mysterious disease that predominantly affects blue-eyed blondes with a light complexion like mine.

On my own, all I could find out about the disease was that the word *lupus* comes from the Latin word for "wolf"; and *erythema,* from the Greek, means literally "to be red." The first thing that came to mind was "What do the wolf and lupus have in common?" The question kept hammering away in my mind. The very sound of the disease was lethal because of its identification with a predator.

MISINFORMATION

Unfortunately, even today, patients read or hear that lupus is invariably a fatal illness; this leads to great anxiety. Physicians observe that when one adds an organic psychosis to these natural fears and anxieties, one gets a hyperirritable, confused person who is afraid of living or dying. Since lupus is a potentially fatal disease, patients suffer from a sense of threatening danger. It's like an apprehension that stays with you even when you have a good day. Always there, it is like a reminder emanating from your blood and cells. It robs you of your peace, and it robs your strength from you. Help with such fears requires much of the physician's time and understanding.

Today, lupus is no longer a rare disease, it is far from being inevitably fatal, and it doesn't predominantly affect blue-eyed blondes. In the United States, African-Americans, Latinos, and Asians have a greater incidence of SLE than Caucasians. (The prevalence among African-American women is estimated by Kaiser-Permanente to be 286 per 100,000 in San Francisco. American Indians are also afflicted by lupus. Sioux Indians have ten times the incidence of lupus as compared with other Native American tribes.

The majority of lupus patients are women (80 to 90 percent). This ratio changes some with discoid lupus (70 to 80 percent are women). The drug-induced type of lupus affects both sexes equally, and close to half of those with childhood lupus are boys.

In 1994, a study conducted by the Lupus Foundation of America, Inc. (LFA) estimated lupus' prevalence nationwide at 1.4 million to 2 million people. While this study cannot replace a detailed epidemiological study, it does provide a credible estimate. It is difficult to establish the correct number of people suffering from this disease because lupus is a collection of diseases. Frequently, medical records indicate that patients have been treated for organ-based problems, but several of these problems may have been manifestations of lupus. Thus, it is possible that many more people have lupus than have actually been diagnosed. In the past twenty years, I have lost several friends to lupus. In each case, the cause of death was recorded as something other than lupus. The complication was listed as the cause of death, rather than lupus itself. All these friends had lupus for many years, but the word lupus does not appear in their obituaries, nor is there any mention that lupus might have contributed to their deaths.

Amazingly, some physicians still maintain that there are only 120,000 people in this country who have lupus. There is a great need for a serious epidemiological study of lupus to establish its prevalence. Unfortunately, nobody is willing to make the necessary investment.

LACKING INFORMATION

There is current increased concern about women's health problems, such as breast cancer, ovarian cancer, diabetes, and the increasing incidence of heart disease in women, but little is being heard about lupus. In 1995, Senator Edward M. Kennedy spoke at Brigham and Women's Hospital in Boston. He pointed out that lupus is a devastating disease. Unfortunately, his voice has been drowned out by prevailing apathy—the same apathy that has prevailed among the majority of physicians for centuries.

I appeared on the same panel with Senator Kennedy and spoke about lupus from a patient's perspective. Here are some excerpts from my speech:

> Lupus is a chronic inflammatory autoimmune disorder that can affect virtually any part of the human body. A normal person produces antibodies to protect against infections, viruses, or other foreign invaders. The lupus patient produces misguided antibodies, which, instead of protecting the person, attack his or her own body's constituent.
>
> Those misguided antibodies can attack the skin, the blood, the kidneys, and they can also affect the brain.
>
> The patient with brain lupus can develop symptoms including depression, inability to concentrate, diminished memory, irritability, personality changes, seizures, psychosis, and other psychological disorders.
>
> Lupus can make a person feel crazy sometimes. This makes me wonder whether many women who are treated for neurosis and are sent home with a handful of Valium are, in fact, lupus patients with brain involvement.
>
> Since I was diagnosed in 1953, some progress has been made in the treatment and diagnosis of lupus. The medications of choice in 1953

were the steroids, and they are still in use. However, today, physicians have learned how to use those potent medications more judiciously, and there are better and more sensitive diagnostic tests. Patients complain that the tests are not yet standardized in all laboratories around the country, and this can cause lots of problems, not only for the patients, but also for the physicians.

To me, lupus remains a disease with a name that is difficult to pronounce and more difficult to live with. It is a disease with an unpredictable prognosis and symptoms that are difficult to explain. It is intermittent and recurrent, and it nibbles away at the will to live and the ability to cope. It can threaten life, and it can prevent the patient from functioning as a normal human being.

The lupus patient is a bewildered person besieged by physical, emotional, and economic problems. The patient becomes ruled by fear—fears that others will find out that one is struck by a mysterious illness, fear of being cut out from the human flow of life, fear of not being able to do the things one was trained to do. One gets worse and then better, without obvious cause. And there are times when the patient is the only person who is sure that they are really sick, but does not know what is wrong.

We need to know precisely what we are suffering from, and we need to know what we are dying of. I feel that our families, our friends, the Social Security office, and our government on whom we rely for funding for research do not understand what lupus is and what it does to a human life.

I feel strongly that, without more understanding, we cannot be properly treated, so we can have a better quality of life and live with dignity and self-respect. We want to look ahead, Senator Kennedy, for more research to find the cause of lupus and find a cure for lupus, which will bring an end to so much suffering and so many unnecessary deaths.

Physicians stress that the past few decades have been an exciting time for research regarding better understanding of the origin and development of lupus and how it affects the body. From the patients' point of view, this is not enough. Patients want to know the cause or causes of lupus, and they want medications with fewer side effects. They stress the need for more public awareness of the disease, more education, and a better understanding not only of the *disease* but also of the *illness* that affects them on a daily basis. Ultimately, they all want a cure and an end to so much suffering and so many unnecessary deaths.

PATIENTS' STORIES

The following is just a sampling of some of the frustrations that lupus patients face, as told by the patients themselves. The first is from the late Emily Heller, a lupus patient who was a physiologist who was actively involved with the Lupus Foundation of America, as she aptly described the lack of understanding of this disease:

At numerous occasions, I have been painfully reminded of the enormous lack of understanding and ordinary knowledge not only on the part of the public sector, but also on the part of medical personnel as well as doctors. The young internists and residents are still sorrowfully lacking in this area. The reason apparently is that there is simply too much to learn and absorb. So the battle for awareness must go on—not only because lupus patients need sympathy and understanding (which, of course, they do), but much more importantly, because of the life-threatening situations that occur regularly within hospitals and clinics because of lack of understanding by both paramedical and medical people.

Another patient writes:

I have no doubt that lupus patients suffer from job discrimination. I speak from first-hand experience, through job hunting and through working in my present position.

While searching for a job two years ago, I honestly "bared my soul" to a prospective employer. I did so partly out of honesty and partly out of self-preservation, as I felt the employer would be more understanding about my absences, although I am in remission and have been for over four years. I might also admit that I thought that having lupus might even be a positive edge (for once!), as the job was health-care related, and I would be classified as a "handicapped female minority."

The employer, who seemed interested in hiring me up until the point of my "confession," suddenly seemed preoccupied, and I did not get the job. Of course, proving this in a court of law would be impossible.

Currently, I am teaching in a suburban high school. Only one close teacher friend there knows I have lupus. Last year, I got bacterial pneumonia, which had no connection to lupus. This year, I got bronchitis. Both illnesses were related to job conditions (no heat). However, when I grieved to the administration, I was very careful not to mention lupus and was terrified they would find out I had it and fire me.

Fortunately, I am healthy now. My classroom conditions are better, and lupus wasn't an issue.

Many people don't know about lupus and may have misinformation, and that may hinder lupus patients seeking employment. Also, since many of us "look normal," it is often not believed we are legitimately ill. Finally, it is very stressful to always worry that every cold, etc., will become a flare and thus reveal the problem.

I have no offers of solutions for the problem, but I certainly wish I could be open about my illness, which among other things, would be a great stress relief to me.

Male patients also have concerns specific to their cases, as this male patient explains:

You talk about self-esteem, ego, morale, value, sexual needs, and how they will affect housekeeping and mothering? Well, let's talk about how it affects men for a change!

How can we keep our wives and children happy and fulfill their needs as well as our own? How do I, as a "broken" man, tell my two-year-old child that Daddy can't play with her, or, quite often, communicate with her because I am too tired to talk, to move, even to think . . .

I've had problems with the medical profession and the Social Security system, probably more so because I am a male and because they lack knowledge about lupus. When I experienced symptoms, I would go from doctor to doctor in search of help, only to be told by each if them, "It's all in your head." This is a diagnosis given to many lupus patients.

Not until a few years ago when my wife rushed me to the emergency department at the hospital, and my doctor put me in the intensive care unit did I start to get minor results. My doctor wanted to give me more antibiotics to lower my blood count, which was quite elevated. I refused to take any additional medication until they read my critique of all my hospital stays. I underlined the high points after my wife typed up four pages condensing my medical history. Then and only then was a proper course of action taken.

It has been one year since I began a steroid program; finally I'm down to prednisone every other day, but I have not had a remission period. I must take quite a bit of medication: Minipress (prozasin hydrochloride)—4 mg daily, lexid—20 mg daily, Tranxene (chlorazepate potassium)—22.5 mg daily, amitriptyline—50 to 100 mg daily, nitroglycerin as needed, Imodium (loperamide hydrochloride) as needed, and Tylenol No. 3 as needed! Plus antibiotics for the constant infections! Drugs and more drugs; that's all they have to prescribe. They leave the rest to the psychiatrists who often have no idea how lupus affects a human life. My resident shrink tells me I handle my disease well, but he's not in my shoes; he's not feeling the emptiness, torment, inadequacies, memory lapses, and stuttering that continues to make me want to withdraw into my own little world!

The most important thing I've learned about this disease is that doctors fill out prescriptions and hand out hefty bills knowing full well you're not covered by adequate insurance. I would love to go back to work as a floor worker in the Chicago Board Options Exchange and regain my vice-presidency title!

HOW LUPUS AFFECTS WORK

Peter Senne is president of MedSafe, Inc., and his wife has lupus. He is a regular contributor to *Lupus Letter,* and has written extensively about improving the workplace for patients with lupus and other chronic illnesses.

Lupus is a devastating diagnosis to its sufferers. In most cases, it changes life as an individual has come to know it. The universal symptom that seems to have this impact is fatigue—inconsistent energy and productivity. Lupus patients can become lacking in control, planning ability, and stamina—hallmarks of organization in home life and business life—from time to time due to fatigue, and adjustment can be difficult.

The operative word in living (and working) with lupus is adjustment. My experience with this adjustment is a personal one. My wife, business partner, best friend, and mother to our four children has taught me about adjustment through her decade of struggle with lupus.

Helping Your Employer Adjust

In order for your employer to know your limitations and offer appropriate help toward your personal adjustment, you must first understand and communicate your needs reasonably and effectively. Although some symptoms, like fatigue, are common to many lupus patients, other manifestations are highly individual and triggered by unique things: food allergens, infection, temperature changes . . . a seemingly endless list. For this reason, even a very general set of recommendations for accommodating lupus patients won't be found in most company policies, or be understood by most employers. Therefore, your first step is to educate.

There is plenty of literature available to assist you in introducing lupus and its possible characteristics to your employer. (Even this book could be your beginning.) An employer needs to be educated about the chronic nature of lupus and its flares and manifestations as they affect you. This can be scary information to share. Your personal views on the confidentiality of your illness and its disclosure to others need also be expressed. Sometimes the special accommodations offered to you will draw the attention of the entire staff, and it's often helpful to eliminate bad feeling, alleviate fears, and even solicit your colleagues' support by educating them, too.

So why would an employer embrace a chronically ill patient with a lupus diagnosis? From a bottom-line perspective (where an employer should rightfully expect productivity), what motivates an employer to pursue these adjustments? Many companies demonstrate a willingness to work with their employees' individual concerns through family-care policies. Employers strive to foster employee loyalty as well as productivity. Flexibility with a chronically ill yet seasoned employee can offer similar rewards.

Making Your Own Adjustments

Functioning with lupus requires you to continue to work and keeping your mind active will minimize your focus on your illness. However, you simply can't do more than your body will allow. Try to devise a work schedule that has you working when you feel strongest. This may mean a four-hour work day, working at home, or working fewer days. Depending on the stage of your lupus and its severity, you may need a temporary leave of absence to respond to your body during its acute phase. Discuss having your work based on productivity, not on hours spent at the desk. Talk with your employer about the best way for you to meet the demand of a forty-hour work week or a part-time schedule. Remember, flexibility must extend both ways. If you expect your employer to be flexible, you must be so, too.

The following adjustments may help to make your work environment productive.

Lighting

Window offices are the envy for some, but not for SLE sufferers. Ask to position your desk far away from any contact with the sunlight, and don't forget those sky-lights! Fluorescent lighting can also be a problem for some.

Temperature

SLE sufferers should be neither too hot nor too cold. Ask to have the heating/air conditioning system balanced frequently. Most companies have an HVAC contract as part of regular maintenance. As a safeguard, see that locks are put on the temperature controls so that only authorized individuals can adjust thermostats. Your employer may also be willing to provide fans and space heaters for your personal use, if necessary.

Comfort

If your job requires long periods of standing, ask for an appropriate chair for occasional breaks. If your position involves bending, lifting, or walking long distances, ask to be transferred or take on other responsibilities that are less physically demanding. Conversely, if your job requires you to sit at a desk all day, make sure your employer knows that you may need to stretch your legs frequently. This may mean taking a five-minute walk every hour or so. Ask your employer to provide a "resting place" where you may lie down to rejuvenate from periodic fatigue. This may mean purchasing a cot and blinds to darken an office.

Self-Help

Be prepared. Make sure you know your limitations and what will rejuvenate your system. Have the proper foods on hand (candy corn) for times when you may need them. Learn to recognize when you need to take a break. Use breathing techniques to relax. If you need to leave work, be prepared to take this as unpaid time.

Stress

First, last, and throughout your day, minimize stress. With any job comes stress, so try to avoid the jobs that are prone to it. Learn to delegate as much as possible and program yourself to really "leave the job at the office" when you go home. If you follow this formula, you may not have to reduce your work schedule to part-time. Keep your work at work!

Ergonomics

Do your wrists hurt when you type on the keyboard? Do you have blurred vision when you turn away from your computer? Does your back get stiff if you sit in your chair all day? It's not that you're getting older—it's more likely that you need to look at the ergonomics, or the positioning, of your work station. Ergonomics is the applied science of workplace equipment design used to decrease worker discomfort, thereby maximizing productivity. Its use can be very important to the lupus sufferer. Ergonomics as a concept can be difficult for some people to understand. Not everyone is savvy in the positioning of computer keyboards, and most offices do not consider ergonomics before setting up work stations. And there is usually little or no training for employees to make them aware of ergonomics risks in the workplace.

Today, ergonomics is gaining ground as a way of preventing workplace injuries. Employers must look at and assess the way people work—including posture, joint angles, and vision. Employees must be aware of the important steps they can take to avoid injury, especially since many workers spend most of their time in front of computers and behind desks.

Guy Fragala, Ph.D., PE, CSP, Director, Department Environmental Health and Safety at the University of Massachusetts Medical Center, Worcester, MA, says "You have to think about work posture in the small office," he says. "Areas to be concerned about are the wrists, elbows, knees, back, neck, and vision." Fragala, one of the leading gurus in ergonomic studies and its impact in the workplace, has identified some risk factors to consider.

Body Positioning

"The optimum position for knees and elbows is a 90-degree angle. This can be achieved through a foot rest or by purchasing a chair that is adjustable so that both knees and elbows are in a comfortable position," Fragala says.

Wrist Posture

A common ergonomic problem is the wrist, which is at risk for repetitive motion injuries, such as carpal tunnel syndrome. When typing at a keyboard, Fragala suggests keeping the wrists in a natural or neutral posture. Hands should be bent up slightly. Wrists and arms should also have support through a wrist rest or other protector.

The Back

"When you're sitting down for long periods of time, you need support in the lumbar section—where your back curves in," Fragala says. This support can be achieved with the correct chair or through other types of back supports, such as specially made back rests or pillows.

The Neck

Look straight ahead when you are sitting and looking at a computer to avoid bending your neck too much, which can lead to injury. Do not look down or peer up at a computer screen.

Vision

A computer monitor should be at arms' length, but there are other factors to consider. If you wear corrective lenses (eye glasses or contact lenses), consider getting glasses just for computer use.

Getting Started

Well, now that you've learned all the benefits of ergonomics, are you wondering how to begin to implement it in your office? Here are a few suggestions for making your workstation ergonomically sound.

Start With an Assessment

Assess your own work habits and workstation with lupus in mind; specifically, which types of actions cause you the most pain or create an uncomfortable working situation. Use this assessment as a jumping off point for bringing your concerns to your employer and developing an overall workplace ergonomics initiative. Determine the changes you can make on your own, such as adjustments to chairs, changing desk placement, lowering keyboard, and so on. Small changes can minimize a person's strain and avoid pressure on key areas of the body.

Record the Number of Times You Do a Task Daily

You need to determine whether a task is repetitive. Decide if a task is done occasionally or daily, if it puts stress on different body parts, and if these tasks are done for longer or shorter periods of the day.

Identify Stressors

Cumulative trauma disorders (like carpal tunnel syndrome) can be caused by stress on the muscles or joints. These stressors can be mechanical or from the force of pushing and pulling. Mechanical stress can be caused by leaning on sharp edges, which may lead to blood flow restriction. Make sure that you are working on a padded surface. Also, avoid lifting and holding, which are two types of stressors.

Check Lighting

Glare is a major contributor to vision problems. Use an anti-glare filter, and position a computer monitor so that it is not in direct sunlight. Do not look directly out the window when you shift your eyes away from a computer screen. Track lighting is also very helpful by placing lighting only where needed.

Check Indoor Air Quality

Your office should regularly check carbon dioxide levels, and make sure there is enough fresh air flow into the office by balancing the heating/air conditioning system. If air vents and ducts are not regularly cleaned or checked, mold and fungi can grow, causing allergic reactions or illness that can further act on your already weakened immune system. Don't forget to consider your carpet as a source for potential allergic reaction, and check to see that the office is cleaned regularly.

Monitor Noise Levels

In the typical office, the photocopier, printers, and other noise makers can disturb hearing or cause hearing problems. Noisy equipment should be placed away from work stations and encased in a separate room, if possible.

Employer Checklist

An employer can prevent workplace injuries by implementing an ergonomics program. However, in order to implement such a program, the employer must ensure that all factors are considered and that workers understand the concept of ergonomics, as well. The following is a checklist to help employers.

- Do you consider the ergonomics benefits when purchasing chairs and furniture for employees?
- Are employees consulted in these purchases or fit to the chairs, desks, or other equipment?
- Do you have a training program for the ergonomically correct way to use the chair or furniture?
- Do you allow frequent breaks during the day?
- Do you assess employees for repetitive motion in their daily routines or tasks?

Employee Checklist

Sometimes when employers implement ergonomics programs, they do not address the needs of all employees. You can help by bringing your concerns to light and offering this checklist for the employers' consideration.

- Are you comfortable in your daily tasks or routine?
- Do you ask for help if you notice risk factors?
- Do you follow the ergonomic advice given to you through training?
- Are you willing to make the changes necessary to protect yourself from repetitive motion injuries?

FATIGUE

Even though lupus affects people in different ways, and one can experience different symptoms, lupus fatigue is something that all of us have in common. The exhaustion remains a symptom that is difficult for patients to explain, and it is not properly understood by the physicians. Many lupus patients, if not all of them, experience an intense fatigue. The lupus fatigue is unique—it absorbs the whole person. It doesn't act like physical or emotional fatigue, or even fatigue that results from other illnesses. It doesn't respond to drugs, rest and relaxation, or psychiatric help. When fatigue results from excessive work, recovery is a matter of time, but prolonged illness leaves patients with a deadly, inexorable tiredness. You feel helpless, as if all the power of recuperation has vanished. Every part of your body feels exhausted. You cannot call it malaise or even lethargy. You feel depleted of energy and spiritually exhausted to the point where brushing your teeth becomes a difficult chore. At times, the sense of futility is so great that one becomes tempted to give up or give in to permanent sleep. What keeps one going is the need to help one's children, attend to a job, or honor the moral responsibility one feels for life itself. Understanding lupus fatigue and its link to depression has become more urgent as observations reveal its damaging effect in many, perhaps in all, patients. Many lupus patients describe this fatigue as their first symptom, and some patients claim that they experience this symptom even when their physicians tell them that they are in remission. Some patients complain that they are exhausted when they get out of bed in the morning, while others experience fatigue in mid-afternoon or evening. Some patients note that rest does not alter their feeling of fatigue. Some believe they feel stronger when they are taking steroids, while others believe the contrary.

A few years ago, in a conversation I had with Dr. Naomi Rothfield, she said:

> Significant fatigue is present in about 85 percent of patients with SLE at the time of diagnosis. In the smaller number of patients who deny the presence of fatigue, the disease may be as severe as in those with significant fatigue. Patients complain that they are exhausted in mid-afternoon, whereas previously they could continue with the usual activities without significant fatigue until after dinner. In other patients, exhaustion may occur even earlier in the day. Some patients note merely that they must go to bed immediately after dinner, whereas previously they could spend the evening with their families or pursue events of interest to them.
>
> The cause of the fatigue is not clear in all patients. Some SLE patients may be severely anemic, while others may have severe renal disease, but these patients are very rare at the time of diagnosis. Patients who run a fever at the time of diagnosis may be exhausted due to the fever. However, the basis for the fatigue in the majority of patients is unknown.

Many physicians believe that the fatigue disappears as the disease goes into remission. In my case, even after years of a complete remission, I still get tired easily, and I can't do as much as I did prior to becoming ill. As I get older, it is difficult for me to ascertain whether my fatigue is age-related or whether I feel tired because I still harbor the predisposition of the disease.

Physically active patients say that they feel better after they exercise, and physicians agree with them. Physicians stress that exercise may lead to less bone loss due to osteopenia induced by corticosteroids, and they recommend walking as a mode of exercise. In areas where winter weather or excessive heat in the summer make outdoor walking impossible, an indoor program of gentle aerobic and muscle strengthening exercises is suggested as a good substitute. As the patient becomes stronger because of exercising, and if there is no medical contraindications, your physician might recommend exercise class to you to take at least three times a week. An exercise program of any sort should not be undertaken without consulting a physician.

In some patients, at some time during the course of the disease, rest rather than exercise may be appropriate. I find that rest helps me a lot, and I find that a healthy and positive attitude toward the disease is very important. A friend of mine, a psychiatrist in California, once told me that a laugh a day is better than an apple a day, and I found him to be right. I learned that it is also useful to learn about your own disease by discussing the presence of any signs of activity with the physicians and learn to recognize the fatigue that is part of the disease.

5

In Conversation With Robert B. Silver, Ph.D.

by Henrietta Aladjem

A year or so ago, on a plane returning to Boston from Atlanta, I fell into a conversation with a pleasant young man who was sitting next to me. In the course of small talk, the young man introduced himself. His name was Dr. Robert Silver and he worked at Woods Hole Marine Biological Laboratory as a research fellow and a teacher for the past twenty-five years. He looked to be much younger than a person who could have done all that.

He mentioned that his primary research interest was the intercommunication within and among the cells, including those in the human body. He believes they speak a "language," which he is trying to decipher. A translation of this, he believes, could make many diseases easier to understand.

I asked Dr. Silver whether I could have been harboring lupus in my cells at that early age, and whether those cells were trying to communicate to me that someday I would develop a severe case of lupus. Dr. Silver smiled and shrugged his shoulders a bit. I asked Dr. Silver whether his research would lead to analyzing human behavior. He said he thought that that might be possible, eventually. I told him about the speculation that Beethoven had lupus. I have always been intrigued with the fact that a composer could write such glorious music, even after he had become deaf. Dr. Silver said he must have written that music in his mind long before he became deaf, and had stored that music essentially within circuits in his brain. It made no difference whether he was deaf or not, he could hear the music in his mind and knew what the music would sound like when played by an orchestra. After a moment of silence, Dr. Silver said, "Mozart produced such a large quantity of music before he died at such an early age. He probably crammed all he could into his short life." Why? Might he have had a feeling, a premonition of his early passing? Perhaps he wanted to be sure that all the important music was written before he died. I mentioned Flannery O'Conner, the Pulitzer Prize winning writer from Atlanta. O'Conner's father had died of lupus. She was told by her physician that lupus did not run in families, yet a few years later she was diagnosed with the disease. Her physician also assured her that she wouldn't die from the disease because of the advances in early diagnosis and treatment. O'Conner finished her last book in the hospital three days before she died. Did she know that she was dying? Did she have a premonition? Following are more important points from my conversation with Dr. Silver.

What Is the Link Between Psychology, Psychiatry, Neuroscience, and Social Science?

Broadly defined, psychology seeks explanations about and treatments for mental breadth and the "mind." Psychiatry is a medical practice that ministers to the mental and emotional needs of the individual. Psychiatric, and, for that matter, psychological, counseling can often be useful for individuals—especially in times of personal need. Neurobiology is the scientific study of the nervous system, ranging from molecules of individual nerve cells through complex, integrated systems, such as the brain. In contrast, the social sciences are focused on studies of the interactions among individuals and groups of individuals, societies, and so forth. Of these four, as a scientist, the neurobiologist is probably considered, by society, to be the most fully removed from the everyday experience.

The overall link between these four disciplines is the mutual effort to understand what can be called our command and control functions exerted through the nervous system, especially as it relates to the sending of, perception of, and response to various types of stimuli.

I have found it curious that we, as a society, so often look askance at a person's seeking counseling from a good psychiatrist or psychologist, but will think nothing of seeking assistance from a dentist for a sore tooth, or a physician for a painful ankle, or, for that matter, a mechanic for trouble with their automobile. Often times, such professionals may help patients see inner strengths, release unnecessary burdens, and provide comfort that complements the comfort sought from family and friends. At these times, such assistance may often be of great benefit.

What Is Premonition?

This is a complex question that goes beyond a few brief comments, and is a somewhat different field from the areas in which I work and study. The bottom line answer is that we do not yet know in a detailed sense what premonition is, other than a sense one gets of things to come, a forewarning, perhaps. Little is understood about what exactly a premonition is; is it real or simply a matter of coincidence?

Let us think of the mind as a set of many pathways that we learn in response to many situations—some simple, some complex. We learn that if we touch a hot pot, it will hurt our fingers. When we see a pot of boiling water on a stove, without touching the pot, we know that our fingers will be hurt if we touch that pot. Since we don't want to hurt our fingers, we decide not to touch the pot of boiling water on the stove. How did we make that decision? We thought of many experiences we have had and, knowing from earlier experience that a hot pot could hurt our fingers . . . and that hurting our fingers is not good for us . . . and that we do not like to feel pain . . . and so on, we find that it is probably best that we not touch that pot of boiling water, lest we injure ourselves. That was a simple situation.

There are many more complex problems that we face each day. Some decisions are based on a nearly complete set of information of which we are aware, like that of the hot pot. Some decisions are made using information we have, but of which we are not consciously aware. Some decisions are made with incomplete information. For example, we are careful when we cross a road—we look in both directions to see if there is an oncoming vehicle. Seeing no automobile coming from the left or right, we assume that we will not be struck by an automobile as we cross the road. While we cannot be certain that an automobile will not travel on the road, we can almost be certain that an automobile will not arrive at the same time as we are crossing the road.

There are many factors we consider: Where is the road? Is it a street in a quiet city neighborhood? Is it a gravel road in the country? Is it a superhighway? What is the time of day? Have we ever had an automobile pass us by at close distance? Have we ever been struck by an automobile? Are we in a hurry to cross the road? There are hundreds of other factors we have to consider when we decide whether or not to cross a road.

Sometimes, we may not have access to any information about a situation, but "know" that "something" is likely to occur. Sometimes we are correct and say that we have had a premonition. We usually ignore those situations in which our guess or "premonition" was incorrect, or believe that we were somehow mistaken.

Is Research Being Conducted to Overcome the Barriers Between Psychology, Psychiatry, Neuroscience, and Social Science?

There are no "barriers," as such, among these fields. Psychology, psychiatry, neuroscience, and what is called social science are distinct disciplines that are generally concerned with how our actions and behavior, which involve various levels of organization of nerve cells—from single nerve cells to groups of nerve cells, to our brain and mind—function. The "barriers" are simply those of delineation. These definitions are much like those for people who would be involved in building a house: a carpenter, a plumber, a painter, a roofer, and so forth. There is research being conducted in each of these areas, and there is research that bridges two or more of these areas.

Will Your Research Help to Understand and Alleviate Panic Disorder?

Not directly. While there may be clues from my work on detecting and characterizing chemical language in living cells that can be applied to such disorders, it is most likely that more closely related studies will provide needed information.

Are We Helpless Against Our DNA?

(As I asked this question, I was thinking of my great-grandmother Heneriette. I told Dr. Silver all about her, and I touched briefly on some of my other ancestors. I told him, "When I look at Heneriette's portrait, the gaze in her eyes is just like mine. It makes me wonder how much of her is living in my cells.")
As our DNA is an essential, integral part of us, we are not at odds with our own blueprint. Each of the 100 trillion cells in your body contains DNA. Each cell contains a small spherical structure called the nucleus, within which resides chromosomes. (That is, with the exception of each of the red blood cells, as they do not

contain a nucleus or chromosomes.) The chromosomes are made up of DNA and protein. That DNA provides the blueprint for each of the cells and tissues and organs of your body. The blueprint has many sets of instructions, or genes, perhaps 20,000 to 30,000 different genes. Each of these genes has the instructions needed for a cell to build one protein, sometimes making many copies of that protein in each cell.

When a cell divides, a process called mitosis, each new cell has the same genetic makeup. That is because before the cell divides, it makes a copy of its blueprint, then sorts the copies of the blueprint so that each new cell has the correct set of information. That process usually works perfectly; however, sometimes it does not. In such cases, the cell does not survive, or it performs improperly. It is the process of how a cell decides to divide that I study in my laboratory.

That blueprint is the product of the mixing of genetic information that occurs when an egg from your mother was fertilized by a sperm from your father. Since an egg contains only half of the genetic information from your mother, and a sperm contains half of the genetic information from your father, that fertilization results in the mixing of the genetic information from your mother and father into the formation of a genetically unique individual—you. Your unique blueprint is read and followed throughout your life by the cells in your body. Those 100 trillion cells act in concert, not against one another—essentially under the control of a government of the body.

When we are well, all is said to be good. When disease is present, it is often due to some instruction on the blueprint that results in a malfunction at the level of the molecules that carry out the chemical reactions necessary for part of the life processes in a cell. Think of those molecules as parts of a clock. If all the parts are present, in working order, in the correct place at the correct time, and being properly regulated by their adjacent parts, then the clock will function properly. If all works well with you, you are said to be in good health. In some situations, if there is an instruction in the blueprint that results in a malfunction, then you may have what we call a disease. In that case, scientists like myself help to define the exact nature and cause of the disease, and determine effective methods for treatment of that condition, and physicians and surgeons help to develop and provide treatment to their patient. So, we are each following our individual blueprint.

Can We Escape Our Genetic Inheritance?

No, it is the blueprint of our genetic makeup.

Can We Predict This Co-Inheritance?

No, the sets of instructions, or genes, in your genetic blueprint were determined by the genes in the chromosomes in the sperm and the egg that became you.

What Is the Relationship Between My Genetic Makeup and That of My Grandmother?

We now know your genetic relationship to your mother and father. Each of them had a similar relationship to their mothers and fathers, and so on. So, some of the genes of your mother, which she received from her mother (your maternal grandmother) were passed on to you. In that case, we would say that you inherited that part of your genetic makeup from your maternal grandmother.

After talking with Dr. Silver, I could feel Heneriette's genes planted even deeper into my cells and soul. It might be fun to pursue in greater detail the other Heneriette's life. It might even help me to take better care of myself.

Late that evening, my daughter, Ingrid, drove Dr. Silver to South Station for him to catch the last bus to Woods Hole. She, too, was fascinated talking with him, and he almost missed his bus because of the lively conversation.

6

Dr. Gerald Rodnan–
A Memorable Encounter

by Henrietta Aladjem

Some years ago, I spoke at a lupus meeting in Pittsburgh, where I met Dr. Gerald Rodnan, a renowned rheumatologist and an exceptionally kind and pleasant person. Dr. Rodnan, who was also one of the speakers at that meeting, commented on the lupus patient's vulnerability to veiled criticism. He said that doctors may involuntarily send the message that this bizarre, poorly understood disease is an annoyance to cope with and treat.

"Inquisitive patients are truly the best patients," he said, "because they challenge physicians and make them aware of the terrible problems associated with having this disease. The best patients are not those who quietly accept what's being done or not being done, but those who want answers to their questions."

In preparation for delivering the presidential address to the American Rheumatism Association, he said, he had looked through the programs of the Association from its inception in Cleveland in 1934. "There were then no papers on lupus on the program," he said. "There was no mention of lupus at all. However, in 1976, fully 30 percent of the papers delivered at the annual meeting of the Rheumatism Association dealt with lupus in one way or another."

Dr. Rodnan predicted that in the near future, physicians will have much more ability to deal with lupus. He stressed the importance of early diagnosis because that is when treatment is most effective. He strongly believed that patients and volunteer groups throughout the country who really give of themselves foster interest in solving many patient problems and increase physician interest in the disease.

A year later, at another lupus meeting in Pittsburgh, Dr. Rodnan invited me for dinner with his family at his house. After dinner, Dr. Rodnan spoke about the history of lupus, about which he was very knowledgeable. He also talked about Roman and Greek mythology and the ancient medical gods, in particular Asclepius and his two daughters, Hygeia and Panacea. Panacea, he said, specialized in the knowledge of medications extracted from plants, and their effects on the body. She was responsible for the curative philosophy of medicine that is so widely accepted today. Hygeia, on the other hand, was concerned with the maintenance of health. She specialized in prevention, and her philosophy lives today in schools of public health, he said.

Asclepius's concept of the practice of medicine was based on the anatomical and physiological knowledge of the time, as well as the beliefs and clinical knowledge learned from treating the sick. "Learning from patients," Dr. Rodnan said with a thoughtful expression, "is the key to opening the minds of physicians.

I told Dr. Rodnan that I'd read a play or a novel in which it was stated that on the moon, they have their own health-care system. "There are no physicians or hospitals on the moon," I said. "One can live there happily ever after as if in a beautiful dream. On the moon, the government supports a person in each house whose job it is to take care of the healthy. They called such a person a *physionom.* "And then I mentioned that the first physionom in my life was my mother. Her observations, experiences, and intelligence allowed her to make a diagnosis, predict a prognosis, and alleviate symptoms. Mother kept me in bed an extra day after an illness to make sure the symptoms had subsided and that I was strong enough to avoid further infections. I laughed a little when I said, "If Mother were alive today and living in this country, she would have been outraged to see how patients are released from hospitals before they are completely well. I know what can happen to lupus patients on cortisone who, after they are released from the hospital too soon, may develop bleeding, new infections, and unforeseen complications." Dr. Rodnan was quiet and slowly nodded his head.

"In winter," I said, "we had no heat in our bedrooms, and the house was constantly aired. Mother believed that infectious agents increased due to stress in life, and she incriminated poor food, lack of sleep, and insufficient rest in the causation of disease, even when it was clear that the disease was infectious. Mother was aware that I was sensitive to excessive heat, to cold, to the sun, to certain foods, to medications, and to mosquito bites. I got headaches from the winds, and turned blue in the cold. And she knew that I had no resistance to infections. Sometimes, her loving look followed me around as if trying to determine what unknown thing her child harbored.

In the cold weather, Mother watched my toes and fingers turn white, then blue, and finally red. She knew they hurt, and she tried to keep me warm. She was always knitting woolen socks and gloves and scarves. When I left for America, she packed a couple of heavy ski sweaters she had made for me to keep me warm while I crossed Siberia on my way to America. I have worn those two sweaters skiing in the Laurentian Mountains in Quebec, Mt. Blanc in Chamonix, and the White Mountains in Maine. I wore them until they turned into shreds. Those sweaters radiated extra warmth because they were imbued with Mother's love for me . . . but only I was aware of it!"

Dr. Rodnan explained that the changing colors of my fingers and toes had a name. "It's called Raynaud's (pronounced ray-nose) phenomenon, a problem that many lupus patients have," he said. "The disease is named after Maurice Raynaud, a French physician who described the symptoms in 1862. The disease involves the small blood vessels of the fingers and the toes and it occurs when one is exposed to the cold. In the cold, the fingers of the patient turn from a deadly white, to bluish, to an angry red. The whiteness is caused by a spasm in the vessels supplying the area, which reduces blood flow. The blueness that follows results from sluggish blood flow through the vessels that are filled with darker, poorly oxygenated blood.

The redness occurs during the overwhelming of the area with blood at the end of the attack, as the body overcompensates with exuberant blood flow."

"When my fingers turned that deadly white, it was sort of scary," I said. "It was as if part of me was dead or dying, even though I knew that it was a transient condition. My husband often had to take my hands into his own to warm them up. Sometimes he blew his warm breath on them to speed up the recovery. Mother had done the same thing when I was growing up. Since my lupus has been in remission, these symptoms appear only once in a great while, but I still wear gloves lined with cashmere in winter, and I often sleep with woolen socks, especially when I sleep with my window open!"

That evening, Dr. Rodnan invited me to speak to his second-year medical school students. "Medical students," he said, "should listen not only to patients with active disease, but also former patients like you." He tried to emphasize the importance of training students to feel comfortable with patients and to view them as whole persons. "Patients are spouses, parents, friends, and employees. Students should think of them as individuals with personal concerns." After a brief pause, he said, "There are things one cannot learn from medical textbooks. One must learn how patients want to be treated. Physicians must learn how to ask the right questions and learn from the answers." Dr. Rodnan wiped some perspiration from his red face and had a sip of water. "Students are very busy in medical school and have no time to think about what it means to live with disease," he said. "They should know more about lupus. There is still very little written about it. Hearing about it from someone who has lived with it for such a long time will be of some help to them and to many physicians who treat lupus patients. I grant you, all lupus patients are not the same, but most of them have common psychological problems and challenges. I have learned a lot from you," he said, looking at me with a winning expression, "but I am sure that I could learn even more by talking with other patients in a relaxed atmosphere without watching the clock. Although we can help the seriously ill patients with lupus, let's not forget that there are thousands and thousands with less severe disease who have a chronic condition and are in need of our care and attention."

Dr. Rodnan's asking me to speak to his medical students was an uncommon practice at the time. Since then, the practice of patients teaching medical students has grown steadily into regular programs at many medical schools throughout the country. Now, patients are part of the regular courses on doctor-patient relationships, and these courses seem to be highly successful.

After my visits to Pittsburgh, I met with Dr. Rodnan several more times in Boston when he attended medical meetings. A few times, I picked him up at the airport where he would arrive late in the evening, looking tired and out-of-breath walking through the airport. He always wore cherry-red socks. I wondered whether those bright socks were something he had loved in his childhood. I should have asked him about that. Perhaps his answer would have allowed me a glimpse into his soul—a glimpse into his goodness. Dr. Rodnan also asked me to join him in speaking to physicians in their continuing education courses in the Pittsburgh area. He also asked me to write a chapter on the "Psycho-Social Problems of Patients with Rheumatic Diseases" for the seventh edition of the *Primer,* a textbook for physicians and medical students.

When I told Dr. Rodnan that I was unfamiliar with the subject and needed his help, he smiled and told me a story about a man who once went to see the French playwright Jean Baptiste Poquelin Molière, who was a master of the French language and known for his wit and charm. The man asked Molière to teach him how to speak in prose; to which Molière replied, "But my dear man, you are already talking in prose, and you don't need any extra tutoring." Dr. Rodnan reassured me, "I'll help you write the chapter, but you'll do all right by yourself." And I did.

Dr. Rodnan was younger than I was, and I was shocked to learn of his sudden death. A few months later Mrs. Rodnan died, too. The Rodnans were gentle, loving people who extended a helping hand to people by lessening their pain and suffering. I shall always remember them with affection, and continue to trust in the goodness of human nature.

Not long after I last saw Dr. Rodnan, Dr. Peter H. Schur asked me to give the "grand rounds" at Brigham and Women's Hospital. "Ordinarily, grand rounds provide an opportunity for the lecturer to show off a bit, to have the spotlight on his or her own intelligence," wrote Dr. Carl Pierce, an old friend of mine, in a book called *The Body Is the Hero* by Ronald J. Glassier, M.D. Unlike neurology rounds or hematology rounds, during which only a few specialists are present, the whole department of medicine comes to grand rounds to listen to what they know will be a definitive discussion of the disease under consideration. The facts are usually presented by a knowledgeable, self-assured expert totally in control of the facts. Sometimes a patient is present to further prove the expert's findings.

I remember trembling with emotion as I stood before some of the top medical scientists and clinicians at Harvard Medical School and Brigham—I had to speak from introspection and personal experience and conversations I had had with other lupus patients. I had no slides to give me a breather. I was the patient, with nothing to rely on except myself.

I could feel the absolute silence around me, and I could see some of the raised eyebrows in the audience. I was grateful to Dr. Schur who sat in the front row and encouraged me with his kindly smile. And I remember telling myself not to waiver or panic. I was there to tell these medical students and practitioners and those studying to become medical practitioners about my thoughts and experiences as a patient, and how much suffering I had to endure.

I told them that I believed that I had a genetic predisposition to the disease. Yet, I did not know of anyone in my family who had anything similar to lupus. Many of my symptoms throughout my growing years were misunderstood. Constant strep throat, susceptibility to cold and heat, recurring pneumonia, and the overreaction to mosquito bites were but a few of the problems, and my mother used to attribute some of my afflictions to a delicate constitution: But father contended that as the only daughter, I was spoiled by everyone in the family and may not have been so sick if I had not been so protected. He had a fundamentalist view of resistance to disease. He never thought of illness as something to spend time on.

I thought in simple terms—strong genes for this, weak genes for that. I fancied a series of barriers, of stages in lupus. Those with the weak genes for resisting lupus would put up a weak defense at each barrier and would get lupus. In this primitive theory, everyone could get the disease if the stimulus was strong enough.

In my case, infections were the beginning—the first barrier. I got too many of them, my defenses were weak, and I needed drugs to help me over the trouble.

The drugs were the second barrier. Instead of helping, they caused new problems which were not interpreted correctly. The reactions should have been gratefully received as a warning signal from nature, not just for one drug but for all. Now, I am even afraid to take aspirin. Yet, for many years, I swallowed new pills and took injections passively, without thinking twice. I should have learned from experience, but along with my physicians, I had to be hit over the head with the allergic reactions many, many times before drawing the right conclusions.

The next barrier in my simple theory occurred when I moved from Bulgaria to Boston where I had to adapt to the water, the food grown with artificial fertilizers, the noises, the lights, the humidity in the summer and in the winter, the dry air in the apartment from the radiators. The stress of being away from home, of having to learn a new language, of working, and of becoming a wife and mother might have helped trigger the lupus. (I have expounded on such thoughts before in *The Sun Is My Enemy* and *In Search of the Sun.*)

My early symptoms, except for the butterfly rash, were so peculiar that they drew attention away from the physical illness. There was no communication among doctors in this ignorance. The pills kept coming, and I willingly took them. The last barriers fell, the disease took hold, and the diagnosis was easier to make. I was lucky. I had good doctors who stuck by me and wanted to help me. I paused for a moment as if to turn to a fresh page in my story and then said, "I am a living example of Osler's old adage: 'If you want to live a long life, get a chronic disease and take care of it.'"

My last sentence brought a few tiny smiles to the faces of my listeners. There were no questions asked and I was relieved that the ordeal was over.

After I finished my talk, I walked back through the old parts of Brigham where my physician of many years Dr. Frank Gardner had his laboratory. I sat on the same old wooden bench by the door where I had waited for the results of my blood tests, and I reflected about then and now.

In the past few decades, there has been much progress gained in research in the fields of immunology and autoimmunity and lupus, but what did the doctors learn about the human condition and how lupus affects a human life? Not much. I question whether one can properly treat the patient without knowing that. Medications and technology can save lives, but a patient needs close human contact with his or her doctor. One needs to exchange thoughts, feelings, and experiences that are hard to handle on one's own.

Such interaction is essential with lupus. The patient needs the comfortable feeling of being able to discuss emotional and psychosocial problems with the physician. The physician has to be informed of all the possible changes with the disease so he or she can be prepared for the unforeseen emergencies. Lupus is an unpredictable disease. Its problems transcend more ordinary medical activities. Scientific knowledge and statistics permit a broad spectrum of knowledge, but there still remain the individual's daily problems.

The thoughts were rushing in my head. That day I was given a chance to talk, and the physicians a chance to listen. My speaking to those doctors was a beginning. Sitting on that bench, I felt like the biblical figure Lazarus whose life was given back to him by divine forces.

In the car on the way home, I reflected some more about the role Dr. Gardner played in bringing about my remission. I think of him as the second physionom in my life.

7

Self-Efficacy and Chronic Disease

by Steven J. Kingsbury, M.D., Ph.D.

Steven J. Kingsbury, M.D., Ph.D., Assistant Professor of Psychiatry at the University of Texas, Southwestern Medical Center, lived in Boston before moving to Texas. Dr. Kingsbury is both a doctor and a patient—he has multiple sclerosis— and he still comes to Boston to see his physicians for an annual check-up. On one of his visits, he took the time to speak to a group of lupus patients about his own experiences with illness. His talk was a major success.

I called Dr. Kingsbury in Texas and talked with him further about his life with multiple sclerosis. He was very pleasant and kind over the phone, and as I got to know him better, I was deeply touched by every word he said. I hope to meet him in person when he comes next time to Boston. Here are some of Dr. Kingsbury's thoughts:

DISCOVERING THE ILLNESS

As someone who is trained both as a psychologist and a psychiatrist, chronic illness has always had some academic interest for me. Unfortunately, I learned more about the topic when I diagnosed myself as having multiple sclerosis (MS) fourteen years ago during my first medical school rotation.

The first sign of my illness occurred when I developed blindness in my left eye, a common symptom of MS. An opthamologist found nothing wrong because the damage was in back of the eye (at least he did not try to imply that psychiatric illness was the cause of my problems). In any case, I was told not to worry and was sent on my way. I decided to read through my medical textbooks and try to find the problem myself. Once I had the likely diagnosis, I arranged for a medical test. My doctors calmly and pleasantly asserted that I was overreacting and that I was just "chasing zebras"—looking for rare conditions when a common condition is probably the cause. With persistence, I persuaded them to perform the necessary tests, and unfortunately, I was proven right. I later learned that it often takes about six years from the first symptom until a diagnosis of MS is made. So I learned early on that I would have to be persistent to get good care, and that my concerns would be minimized by doctors who depreciate the problems of others.

Since the time I was diagnosed, I have learned many lessons, such as how to handle condescending doctors who don't take my condition seriously. Some of the most important lessons, however, have to do with the need to maintain a sense of self-efficacy—the sense that I control my own life in many ways, not just in relation to my MS and its treatment. This reflects my understanding of how psychology can affect my relationship to my disease, how I've learned to live with that disease at times, and at other times, to live without MS.

FORDYCE'S LAW

I often think of Wilbur Fordyce, a psychologist who has spent his life working with people who suffer chronic pain from such conditions as back injuries. For his achievements in this field, he won an award from the American Psychological Association, and in his acceptance speech, he reduced his life's work to a principle that he called "Fordyce's Law"—"People suffer less when they have something better to do." Although he proposed this law for chronic pain patients, I have found it very helpful for me and even for many severely mentally ill people.

What this means is that I suffer less when I'm doing things for myself—preferably enjoyable things but, nevertheless, activities that I believe are of some importance to me. As an example, I notice chronic tingling in my extremities less when I'm engaged in almost any activity that occupies my mind and needs my attention. When I am writing about it—as I am now—it comes to the forefront of my mind, I become more aware of it, and I suffer with it, but most days, I cannot recall a time when I even noticed my ever-present tingling. Most of the time, I'm too busy for my MS, although I do schedule it in when I have treatments or the blood tests related to them.

It helps that my favored activities are within my present and (hopefully) future capabilities. First, I have a sedentary profession. Second, many of my favorite diversions, such as reading and watching television, are also sedentary. Other activities, like going to the mall, need a little planning, but are not too difficult even with the difficulty of walking. To make sure that I am not too much of a couch potato, I exercise (less than I should) at home, where I can both pace myself and regulate the temperature. I guess I was lucky that I never enjoyed athletics, but if I had, I would be developing other enjoyments within my present capabilities.

DEAD MAN'S RULE

Fordyce's Law is one of the two principles I apply to myself and use with all my patients. The second principle is known as the "Dead Man's Rule," which states that one should never have as a goal of therapy something a dead man can do. For example, a goal of having a child not talk in class would be unacceptable, since a dead man could easily achieve the goal of not talking in class. This leads to the extremely important question of what you would rather have the child doing other than talking in class. One can note that the goals, therefore, are more than just the absence of a problem. The presence of something positive is needed. In many ways, this is related to the goal of people suffering less when they find something better to do.

FACTORS THAT HELP SELF-EFFICACY WORK

Let me add that I have tried to read about my condition and the treatments available. I have tried to affiliate myself with the best doctors I could find. After getting explanations of the treatments, I am very good about following my doctor's treatment plan if I believe it is helping me, even though I might find it very unpleasant. I go back to Boston twice a year to stay in contact with my neurologist, who is one of the leading MS researchers in the world. In other words, I am not denying that I have MS or that I am a patient—it's just not the focus of my life. Most days, my MS does not come up.

Let me also add that I have terrific support, which is extremely important for anyone with a chronic illness. My wife keeps me honest by not helping me when I just want to be lazy, but by being supportive when I need help. Support gives me feedback when I need feedback, a push when I need a push, and some help when I need to modulate stress. Typically, one cannot do it alone. Having a chronic illness can be too much to face alone.

To put what I've said differently, I believe I've structured my life to maintain a sense of self-efficacy—that I can accomplish what I want. Self-efficacy is composed of two parts. First is the belief that your behavior can lead to consistent positive outcomes, and second is the belief that you are capable of producing those behaviors. Again, it is a good thing that I don't want to win the Boston Marathon, so what I do value and want is within my reach even with MS.

According to research conducted on the subject, the sense of self-efficacy confers certain benefits. First, it means that I function under less tension, since I am doing things I believe I can do. Although the link between stress and exacerbation of illness in MS or lupus is unclear, what evidence does exist suggests that being under stress is not desirable—especially when the stress is negative. Relaxation may be helpful for minimizing the stress and is clearly enjoyable. It is also not enough to manage my illness.

Becoming more of a problem-solver is also important. I don't want life stresses to mount without my feeling that I am taking active steps to ameliorate my situation. This does more than simply make me feel good about myself. Increasing evidence suggests that it also helps boost my immune system to help it regulate itself more effectively. This may sound paradoxical, since my immune system is what got me into trouble in the first place, but it turns out that lymphocytes, the main component of the immune system, come in many different types. Some attack what are considered foreign substances, and it is these types of lymphocytes that lose their bearings in autoimmune diseases like MS and lupus. This leads to cells attacking and destroying things they should recognize as part of us. But there are also other cells that modulate the immune response, limiting the action of these harmful cells.

ELIMINATING THE EFFECTS OF STRESS

The body has many checks and balances. We are beginning to understand links between these modulatory lymphocytes and stress. The lowering of stress may aid in the body's modulatory efforts by increasing the numbers and the efficacy of these lymphocytes to hold the destructive ones in check. In other words, being able to handle stress well—with self-efficacy—may act to slow down or prevent autoimmune diseases from advancing as quickly. Like lupus, MS can progress at any speed, from very quickly to very slowly. And, like those with lupus, they tell those with MS to avoid stress as much as possible.

That sounds great, but welcome to the twentieth century! The question is not whether you can avoid stress (because that is almost impossible to do), but how are you going to manage it and not be overwhelmed by it. The first step is recognizing it. This is best done by recognizing situations that characteristically lead to stress as well as by recognizing typical reactions to stress you usually have, like frequent headaches. Once you have recognized that you are under greater stress and hopefully have identified the cause, you have a chance of reducing it by fixing the situation.

Now that sounds easy: You find the source of stress and work to reduce it. Unfortunately, this works only for some sources of stress. Others are not so easy to fix. For the more difficult situations, there are several possible solutions. First is what I mentioned already, using relaxation and other calming techniques. Things often appear less bleak when one is calmer. A second technique for handling stresses that are not readily reducible is to try to maintain your sense of perspective—this means reframing the stressor to see it from another vantage point. I am not necessarily saying that every cloud has a silver lining, but I do mean that most situations can be viewed from more than one perspective. These other perspectives can sometimes give you a handle on how to help at least part of the situation, and doing that can create a more favorable climate for you. Besides, my medical training has taught me—"When in doubt, consult someone else." Others can often see things from a different perspective than I can.

Finally, let me say something about the so-called "courage" of those coping with chronic illness. I once saw a TV interview with a woman with muscular dystrophy who had to stop working because of her condition, but who was, nevertheless, staying as engaged, active, and productive as she was able to.

When the interviewer called her courageous, she somewhat disdainfully replied by asking what else was she supposed to do? She had not chosen to have muscular dystrophy, nor did she have any other choice but to try to make the best of her present situation. Calling people with chronic diseases courageous is, in my opinion, pretty stupid. We're doing the best we can with the cards that were dealt us, just like most people. That neither requires sympathy nor false idealization.

Although it is important for everybody, maintaining and enhancing one's sense of self-efficacy is doubly important for those of us with chronic diseases. Picking the arenas where we can successfully compete is the art of living.

PART THREE

Lupus in Different Facets of Life

Lupus in Different Facets of Life
by Henrietta Aladjem

Though lupus is most common in women, it can also affect men, children, and the elderly. Changes in a woman's life, such as pregnancy and menopause can also affect one's lupus. Information about lupus in special cases is important, since generally, when one reads about lupus, one only reads about the typical cases. Information about lupus is important. It is only through education that we can help to empower the patient. One can deal with the disease more efficiently if he or she is better informed. I hope that this part of the book will help achieve this goal.

Neonatal Lupus
by Michael D. Lockshin, M.D.

When lupus complicates pregnancy, one of the things that frightens prospective and new parents most is the thought that their child might have the mother's disease. Parents who have heard of a condition (wrongly) called *neonatal lupus* often imagine that terrifying things might happen to their child. Most of the time they need not worry. The facts, as they are understood, are as follows:

- Neonatal lupus is very different from systemic lupus erythematosus; it does not develop into SLE.
- Neonatal lupus is rare.
- In most cases, neonatal lupus is not serious and does not need to be treated.
- In most cases, neonatal lupus disappears spontaneously in a few weeks, leaving no after-effects.
- With a blood test, it is possible to tell which women will *not* deliver a child who will develop neonatal lupus.
- Many children with neonatal lupus are born to mothers who do not have SLE.

WHAT IS NEONATAL LUPUS?

The term is used to describe three major symptoms found in newborns. The most common symptom is a rash. The rash can take many forms, but is usually scattered over the body, not necessarily just on the face. It shows up a few days or weeks after birth, particularly after sun exposure, and usually disappears after a few more weeks, leaving no scar. The rash looks like many other rashes that babies get. It can be identified definitively only by biopsy, but this is usually not necessary, since there is little that can be done for the rash, other than waiting for it to disappear.

The second most common symptom is an abnormal blood count: low levels of platelets, anemia, and other abnormalities. Again, this is seldom serious; these abnormalities usually go away in a few weeks with no treatment.

The rarest abnormality, but a serious one, is a heart rhythm abnormality known as congenital heart block. A normal heartbeat starts in the upper heart (the atria or auricles) and travels smoothly through to the bottom of the heart (the ventricles). In heart block, the atrial beat (which generally occurs about 140 times per minute in a newborn) cannot get through to the ventricles because scar tissue blocks its path. The ventricles then have to beat on their own (about sixty times per minute in a newborn). Since the ventricle beat determines the pulse, the baby has an abnormally slow pulse.

Congenital heart block can often be diagnosed between the fifteenth and twenty-fifth week (or the fourth to sixth month) of pregnancy. If the unborn baby has heart block but appears to be doing well, either nothing is done, or a special form of cortisone is given that will go through the placenta to the baby, but it may not make the heart beat normally again. If the baby is not doing well and is big enough to deliver (thirty weeks into pregnancy or later), delivery is often the best way of handling the problem. After birth, many babies with congenital heart block lead normal lives with no treatment, but some need pacemakers, and a small number die from heart disease.

Neonatal lupus is not the same as adult lupus. Babies with neonatal lupus do not develop arthritis, fever, or kidney or brain disease.

HOW CAN RISK BE PREDICTED?

One of the startling recent findings about neonatal lupus is that essentially all mothers of infants with neonatal lupus have a specific set of antibodies. The antibodies are those called anti-Ro (also called anti-SSA) and anti-La (also called anti-SSB). Only about one-third of all lupus patients have these antibodies. The mother who has neither anti-Ro nor anti-La antibodies (about two-thirds of all lupus patients) has no chance of delivering a child with any manifestation of neonatal lupus. The mother who has anti-Ro but not anti-La antibodies has about a 25-percent risk of delivering a child who will develop rash or blood abnormalities. Those women who have both anti-Ro and anti-La antibodies are at highest risk for delivering a child with congenital heart block, but even so, most women with both kinds of antibodies have normal children. (It is very rare for a woman to have only anti-La and not anti-Ro.) If a woman has already had one child with neonatal lupus, the risk that her next child will develop the illness is only about 25 percent.

Many women who deliver children with neonatal lupus do not have symptoms of lupus. In fact, except for their abnormal blood tests, many are well. Looking at the question the other way, no specific characteristics of the illness (except the antibodies) of the mother already diagnosed with lupus changes the risk of neonatal lupus. Lupus patients who are sick are no more nor less likely to have a child with neonatal lupus than lupus patients who are well.

WHAT HAPPENS TO THE AFFECTED CHILD?

It would be nice to give a definitive answer to this question, but because the anti-Ro and anti-La antibody tests have been widely available for only a short time, and because the diagnosis of neonatal lupus has been easily made for only about a decade, long-term observations have not yet been made. Most of the children and adolescents born with neonatal lupus, however, appear to have developed normally. Doctors who have studied them say that they have no higher risk of developing SLE than does any other close relative of a lupus patient. Those with heart disease need to see cardiologists because many will eventually need pacemakers or other treatments.

ARE THERE ANY SPECIAL WAYS TO MANAGE A LUPUS PREGNANCY TO PREVENT NEONATAL LUPUS?

To date, there is no known way to prevent neonatal lupus, but risk can be defined. All pregnant lupus patients can be tested for anti-Ro and anti-La antibodies. Women who test negative can be reassured. They will not have a child with neonatal lupus. Those who test positive for only the anti-Ro antibody should be alerted about the possibility of rash and blood test abnormalities in the child, but should not worry unduly. The pediatrician, and the patient, should not to panic. (Pediatricians are often unfamiliar with neonatal lupus.) For pregnant women who have both anti-Ro and anti-La antibodies, periodic checks on the baby's heartbeat (fetal echocardiography), especially between the fifteenth and twenty-fifth weeks of pregnancy, will identify unequivocally whether or not the baby's heart is normal. If the heartbeat is normal, there is no further worry once the baby is born. If any abnormality does occur, the best available obstetric/perinatal/cardiological options should be obtained, since treatment of this condition requires special skill.

9

Lupus and Kids

by Malcolm P. Rogers, M.D.

Systemic lupus erythematosus poses special problems for children and adolescents. Children have difficulty dealing with the pain; the interruption of normal activities, such as school and sports; the limitation of mobility; change in appearance; and the feeling of being different. Their illnesses may also interfere with normal developmental processes, such as the gaining of social and academic skills, formation of identity, and development of independence and separation from parents.

Children's concepts of disease are rather concrete—generally, based on notions of accidental injuries or catching germs. The more abstract reasoning required to understand lupus does not usually fully develop before adolescence. So, how do you explain to a kid that lupus is a disturbance in the immune system, triggered by multiple factors that range from genetic to environmental factors? Children are focused on the immediate effects and consequences of their disease, such as whether or not they can play their favorite sport today, whether or not they can go out with their friend in the afternoon, or whether or not the disease will go away. It's not until adolescence that children begin to understand the way in which their disease might interfere with their future career or relationship goals, and this may lead to depression.

THE IMPACT ON PARENTS

For parents, the impact of a chronically ill child can be no less monumental. Their emotional reactions are often intense. In today's world, both parents often work and are likely to face time and financial constraints already. It may also take special restraint to not overprotect their ill child. They may fear that they've passed on genetic vulnerability and thus feel guilt. Or they may feel guilt for other reasons that have little to do with the actual development of lupus. After all, both parents and children expect, often unconsciously, that parents will be all-protective. When a child becomes seriously ill, this notion can be shattered. The loss of such a belief can cause fear in the child and guilt in the parent. Parents often struggle to balance the special needs of their ill child with the equally compelling needs of their other children. It may be necessary at times to treat them differently from their siblings, or excuse them from chores or other normal tasks, yet it is important to maintain as much normalcy as possible.

MANAGING LUPUS IN CHILDREN

Lupus in children is essentially the same disease as that which occurs in adults. Some newborn infants of mothers with SLE experience heart defects or temporary skin lesions—the so-called "neonatal lupus syndrome." This is not true lupus resulting from biological disturbances originating in the child. This illness is due to the presence of anti-Ro (SSA) antibodies in the infant's serum, which degrade and disappear gradually during the first year of life. In true childhood lupus, joint pain appears to be the most common complaint, and fever, fatigue, and a butterfly rash are also common. As with adults, kidney involvement is one of the more serious manifestations of lupus. Laboratory abnormalities are similar. The way lupus affects other organ systems is also similar to adults. Peak incidence of lupus occurs near the time of puberty, suggesting a hormonal influence on the onset of lupus in children.

In most parts of this country, children with lupus are treated by pediatricians, and often by rheumatologists with special training in pediatric care. Generally, by the time patients reach adolescence, their care is transferred to an adult rheumatologist, as there are many very competent rheumatologists available who are familiar with the treatment of lupus. However, the timing of this transfer may vary considerably. Patients whose care begins in a pediatric or children's hospital setting may continue their care there—long into their twenties and sometimes into their thirties.

The major difference in managing lupus in children has to do with the special developmental needs of children with illness: their academic growth, moral growth, peer relationships, and emotional maturation. Perhaps the strongest argument for the involvement of pediatricians or pediatric rheumatologists is that they are generally much more attuned to these issues than adult-focused practitioners. They know when, what, and how to communicate with parents, school administrators, teachers, and summer camps. They know how to gently begin to allow more autonomy with adolescents, and to allow parents access to, but not too much control of, their children's health care. They are usually proficient at communicating with children and adolescents, knowing that they need to be warmer, more open and revealing of themselves, and more deliberate in creating an atmosphere where kids feel comfortable and open.

Another significant difference with lupus in children has to do with the effects of certain treatments. For example, prednisone and other corticosteroids can inhibit growth, so steroid use is limited to potentially life-threatening complications, such as renal or brain involvement. Naturally, medication dose is adjusted for the patient's size. When children are treated with corticosteroids, calcium and vitamin D supplementation are used prevent future problems with osteoporosis.

MOVING FROM PEDIATRIC TO ADULT CARE

Transfer to adult treatment settings should occur when patients are medically and psychologically stable. There is less urgency for transfer if the adolescent patient has developed a more grown-up and responsible role in the treatment of his or her own illness. At the beginning of the illness, parents are intensely involved in choosing the doctor, acquiring information, asking questions, and presenting symptoms. Over time, the adolescent patient should assume an increasingly autonomous role in his or her own health care. They should be expected to do the talking and have answers directed to them. They should gain responsibility for handling their medications and scheduling their appointments. They also have a right to confidentiality, which should be respected.

Sometimes transfers to adult treatment settings occur because of natural transitions. The doctor or patient's family is moving. Sometimes the patient is going away to college. Nowadays, transfers occur more frequently when health insurance plans change, and the new plan covers only certain providers or hospitals. Families need to be educated purchasers of health insurance plans, and aware of the complications of restrictions of choice and specialty health care. Sometimes, patients switch to an adult treatment setting because they or their families are unhappy with the care they are receiving, or want a second opinion.

Even under the best of circumstances, children may find such transitions difficult for a number of reasons. First, they are leaving one doctor or set of providers for unknowns. If they have become attached to their doctor, the transition will be experienced as a painful loss. They had become used to a certain *modus operandi,* and now the rules may change. For kids in this transition, new doctors should avoid immediate changes in medications and other routines of care. Patients need to get used to the new doctor and develop some trust first. Moreover, the implicit message in immediate changes may be that what the former doctor did was wrong, and that may, in their eyes, discredit the former doctor, whom they have come to trust.

A second reason a transition from doctor to doctor may be difficult is that they may have harbored thoughts that their disease would go away or that they would outgrow it. Now, they are confronted with the reality that even as they grow up, they are not leaving this disease behind them. Rather, they are faced with this as a chronic and lifelong problem, even if it goes into a prolonged remission. Of course, they may have been told the truth, but denial is a frequent and useful defense, punctured only by confronting such external realities.

One of the biggest issues in the psychological management of children with lupus, or any chronic illness, is to allow them gradually increasing autonomy in their own health care. Adolescents are generally in the process of separating from their parents. They need to see their doctors alone, at least for part of each visit. They need to ask the questions themselves, and gradually assume more responsibility for being in charge of their own medications, etc. They need to begin to feel some control over aspects of their own care—when and where their office visits are scheduled, and ultimately, with whom. A new system for dealing with all of these complicated, often subtle and implicit aspects of their health care will need to be found.

As much as kids want to become independent from their parents, they are anxious about taking these steps, whether it be going away to college, communicating directly with their doctors, making appointments, or generally assuming responsibility for this aspect of their lives. They may forget to take their medicine. They may forget appointments. Sometimes, they do not get necessary rest and sleep. These are opportunities to provide additional guidance, reminders, and encouragement, not to usurp control of their health care. They are also good opportunities for more open dialogue about the issues of independence and expectations of support.

The transition from one doctor to another may also mean the loss of a natural support group of kids their own age who have lupus. There may also be a feeling of loss of the nurse, receptionist, physical therapist, or other people in the former setting. The sense of differentness and isolation that lupus may cause a teenager to feel is especially difficult. It is very important that they have a chance to talk with patients their own age, or somewhat older, who have experienced similar fears and other emotions. The transition into an adult rheumatology practice may be eased by appropriate peer support, perhaps through a local Lupus Foundation chapter. Feeling understood can relieve a major portion of the burden of this illness.

Kids benefit from having some contact with adults who have had lupus and yet manage to live full and gratifying lives. One patient, Vickie Croke, now a journalist for the *Boston Globe,* has written about the importance of discovering the example of Henrietta Aladjem. When Vickie was quite ill as a teenager, she lost hope in ever being able to achieve her vision and goals for adulthood. When she met "Hennie," whose disease by then had been in remission for many years, Vickie's hope was restored. Kids, above all, need a vision for themselves in the future, and adult role models to help provide it.

Fortunately, children and adolescents are extremely resilient. With the support of their family, friends, and doctors most manage to negotiate these extra challenges imposed by their illness. Sometimes counseling or psychotherapy can be very helpful as well. Sometimes, parents need some type of counseling more than their children do. If more persistent difficulties with depression or anxiety arise, psychiatric intervention and referral are appropriate.

10

Lupus in Women

by Naomi Rothfield, M.D.

Lupus affects many more women than it does men. There are at least nine females with systemic lupus erythematosus (SLE) for every male with the disease. In our analysis of lupus patients, we noted that among young children, the proportion of boys to girls with lupus was much closer than it was among adolescents and young adults. In childhood there were only two to three girls for every boy with SLE. When we looked at the elderly, we also found proportionately more males with SLE.

Although SLE does occur occasionally in children and in the elderly, it is mainly a disease of young adolescents and young adults. The disease generally occurs after the onset of menstrual periods. It is much less common prior to menarche and less common after menopause. Thus, the onset of the disease certainly relates to the presence of female hormones, such as estrogen.

Some physicians have reported that estrogens can make the disease worse in patients who start taking supplemental estrogen after the onset of menopause. Other physicians disagree. There is now a large trial of estrogens in post-menopausal lupus patients, which is being funded by the National Institutes of Health. Patients will be given either a placebo (a harmless sugar pill) or estrogen. Neither the patients nor the physicians will be aware of the actual content of the pills that the patient receives. After all the patients have completed the trial, researchers will determine who took the placebo and who took the estrogen. The number of flares that occurred in those taking the placebo and those taking estrogen will be compared. This exciting study should settle the question of estrogen's role in worsening lupus in postmenopausal patients. A similar study by the same group currently underway is testing the role of oral contraceptives in causing flares of the disease in women of childbearing age. These two important studies may help to determine the role of the female hormones in the cause of the disease.

Women have lower levels of male hormones (androgens) in their bodies. A study was done at Stanford University to determine whether a mild androgen pill will improve lupus symptoms in female patients. Dehydroepiandrosterone (DHEA) is a weak androgen that is produced in the adrenal glands, testes, ovaries, and brain. DHEA is also a precursor for several other hormones in the body. It is first converted into DHEA sulfate (DHEAS), the most abundant circulating adrenal steroid in humans. DHEAS is then converted into androgens, such as testosterone, and, to a much lesser extent, into estrogens. Low levels of DHEA and DHEAS have been found in female lupus patients. In lupus mice, androgens have long been found to have a beneficial effect on the disease. DHEA has also been found to affect the immune response, which, of course, also plays a role in lupus. DHEA is now being tested in a large trial to determine whether it may play a role in improving lupus.

These are very exciting times—we have three different studies in which SLE patients are being tested for their response to female hormones (estrogen) and to a weak male hormone (DHEA). It is hoped that within a few years we will be in a position to modify the treatment of SLE with the use of these hormones.

11

Men With Lupus

by Michael D. Lockshin, M.D., F.A.C.P.

"**W**hen writing about lupus, why don't they ever write about men?"

I have heard that question often enough that it might have occurred to me to volunteer to write something myself, but it did not, so Mrs. Aladjem volunteered me instead. I think there are two basic reasons why "they" don't write about men: thoughtlessness on the part of my colleagues and me, and there is not a whole lot to say. For the first reason, I apologize. Sexism, it seems, works in both directions. However, there isn't much conclusive information on any differences in the way lupus affects men and the way it affects women, though only about 10 percent of lupus patients are men.

Antiphospholipid antibody syndrome consists of recurrent blood clots (such as strokes, or clots in the veins of the legs) and in women recurrent miscarriages, associated with anticardiolipin antibody or lupus anticoagulant—together these antibodies are called antiphospholipid antibodies. The syndrome can occur either by itself (primary) or in patients with lupus (secondary). About one-third of patients with lupus have the antibody, but only about one-tenth to one-fifth have the syndrome. Studies differ in details, but some say that men with lupus have more problems with blood platelets, blood vessel blockage, and lung scarring than do women. Prognosis is about the same in men and women. There may be a higher likelihood of disease in a second family member if the first affected member is male. As far as I can tell, men with antiphospholipid antibody truly differ from women in only two ways: they don't get pregnant, so they don't have problems with pregnancy (or with fathering children), and the first doctors they see (in the armed forces, in student health centers) do not believe them when they say their positive tests for syphilis must be false. (A false positive tests for syphilis is a common indicator of both antiphospholipid antibody syndrome and lupus.) As a result, they get treated with penicillin more than do women patients.

Because mouse lupus can be improved by removing the ovaries in female mice, and thus removing the source of female hormones, and can be made worse by administering female hormones, there has been much speculation about how "manly" men with lupus and antiphospholipid antibody syndrome really are. As I see it, they are perfectly normal males. Specific measures of hormone levels in men with lupus have given all sorts of confusing results. As far as observable characteristics go, men with lupus and antiphospholipid antibody syndrome look and act like "normal men": They have normal voices, hair patterns, muscles, sexual drive and performance, fertility, and other "typically male" characteristics. Homosexuality is no more common among patients with lupus and antiphospholipid antibody syndrome than it is among the population as a whole. Furthermore, although some years ago there was a flurry of interest in one clinic that saw several men who had both lupus and a rare, feminizing chromosome abnormality known as Klinefelter's syndrome, most other clinics have not, and the observation has not explained much about male lupus. The bottom line is that men with lupus, except for their disease, are pretty normal.

Some doctors have tried to treat female lupus patients with male hormones. There is current interest in treatment with dehydroepiandrosterone (DHEA—a precursor for some male hormones). Results of studies with the hormone are mixed, even in men. The drugs that cause sterility in women also cause sterility in men. While there is much discussion about the wisdom of giving postmenopausal estrogen to women, I don't know of any significant research on giving testosterone to older men or to men who have been treated with cyclophosphamide.

A fair question is: "Should men and women with these diseases be viewed differently?" The answer, in typical doctor double-speak, is both yes and no. No, because, as far as we know today, the symptoms and the treatment for both men and women are the same. Yes, because any disease with such a high incidence rate for one gender must have an explanation that is important, and yes, because the needs of women and men differ. Thank you, my patients, and thank you, Mrs. Aladjem, for asking.

12

Lupus and the Elderly

by Michelle Petri, M.D.

When I speak of lupus in the elderly, there are actually two groups of people to whom I am referring—those who develop lupus for the first time after the age of fifty, and those who developed the illness earlier in life but are now elderly. Although the great majority of systemic lupus erythematosus patients have their first signs and symptoms in their teens, twenties, or sometimes thirties, it is well known and accepted that a few patients present symptoms for the very first time after the age of fifty. However, drug-induced lupus—which is really a separate disease, with a different genetic predisposition—generally occurs in an older population, because the drugs that cause it, including procainamide, hydralazine, and isoniazid—are more commonly prescribed for the middle-aged and elderly population.

CHARACTERISTICS OF LUPUS IN THE ELDERLY

No center conducting research has large numbers of elderly patients with new onset lupus. This has limited the study of systemic lupus in the elderly. However, certain themes repeat in many of the published studies. There seems to be less of a female predominance in older-onset lupus. Another important finding is that elderly-onset lupus often includes symptoms and signs of Sjögren's syndrome—the dry eye, dry mouth syndrome. Younger SLE patients can also have Sjögren's syndrome, but Sjögren's antibodies, anti-Ro and anti-La, are found more frequently in late-onset SLE.

SLE in those over the age of fifty is generally milder, with more serositis (pleurisy and pericarditis) and arthritis, and less renal and central nervous system (CNS) disease than usually occurs in lupus in the general population. However, not all series have agreed, in that one group found a poorer prognosis for their elder SLE group. There are always exceptions, and some of our sickest lupus patients have been those in which onset occurred after the age of fifty. One problem that may lead to this phenomenon of elderly lupus patients being so sick is that physicians often do not consider SLE as a diagnosis in an elder patient with fever, CNS changes, or pericarditis, which can lead to delay in diagnosis and treatment.

It is truly one of the success stories of the treatment of SLE that young patients are now surviving and becoming elderly! The patients who were diagnosed in the

1970s and 1980s have benefited from better SLE treatment, better antibiotics, and the availability of dialysis and transplantation for kidney failure. Patients diagnosed in the 1990s will also benefit from the vigor that rheumatologists now employ in preventing damage from high-dose corticosteroids. However, keeping this generation of surviving SLE patients healthy is an ongoing challenge, as over 50 percent of surviving lupus patients over the age of fifty have had one or more organ systems permanently damaged by the SLE or its treatment.

CARDIOVASCULAR DISEASE RISK

All elder SLE patients need to be concerned about atherosclerosis and the risk of coronary artery disease and stroke. The best time to begin to be concerned is while in your twenties and thirties, when attempts—both through lifestyle changes and prescription medicines—to reduce cardiovascular risk factors should begin. There is more and more evidence that reduction of cardiovascular risk factors from young adulthood onwards is effective. No longer do physicians want to wait until the patient is middle-aged to begin risk-factor reduction efforts. The major cause of death—and one of the major causes of damage in lupus patients over the age of fifty—is atherosclerosis. Patients with lupus get atherosclerosis earlier than those in the general population, and more frequently. The disease itself may initially damage the blood vessels through inflammation, but if the cardiovascular risk factors are present, the vessel may be more likely to heal with narrowing and atherosclerotic changes.

Research from the Framingham Heart Study identified the major risk factors for heart disease in the general population. These include hypertension, hyperlipidemia (high cholesterol and high LDL cholesterol), smoking, obesity, and lack of exercise. Patients with lupus and severe kidney involvement are more likely to have high blood pressure and lipid abnormalities. However, high blood pressure, weight gain, and high cholesterol are all aggravated by chronic prednisone use (especially when the dose is greater than 10 mg daily). Many patients with lupus may find it difficult to exercise due to joint problems and fatigue, but it is important that the physician, physical therapist, and patient work together to find an appropriate exercise regimen to preserve muscle function and health.

LUPUS AFTER MENOPAUSE

There is a common misperception that lupus does not flare after menopause. Our research shows that lupus continues to evolve, causing new symptoms and signs in new organ systems, in all age groups. Thus, even older lupus patients need ongoing careful clinical and laboratory surveillance to determine the activity of their diseases and to make appropriate treatment decisions.

Estrogen Replacement Therapy

One issue for the postmenopausal patient with SLE is whether or not she should undergo estrogen replacement therapy. For many years, the answer was "no" because of concern that the estrogen would cause the lupus to flare. However, postmenopausal estrogen replacement therapy uses much less estrogen than the amount used in oral contraceptives. In addition, researchers compared groups of lupus patients who underwent estrogen replacement therapy with groups that did not. They did not find any increase in disease flares with estrogen replacement therapy. However, these findings must be tempered by the results of the Nurses Health Study in which nurses who took postmenopausal estrogen seemed to be more likely to develop lupus.

In addition, there has been concern that women with lupus who make antiphospholipid antibodies (including the lupus anticoagulant and/or anticardiolipin antibody), which are associated with an increased risk of blood clotting, might be at greater risk of clotting problems if exposed to estrogen. Overall, however, the benefits of estrogen therapy probably outweigh the risks. Estrogen replacement therapy helps to prevent osteoporosis (for which a woman is especially predisposed if she undergoes any corticosteroid therapy) and helps to reduce the risk of atherosclerosis by maintaing a better lipid profile. In the general population, studies have also suggested that estrogen replacement therapy may help to preserve cognitive function and prevent osteoarthritis.

Because of the importance of estrogen replacement therapy and ongoing concerns about its effect on disease activity and clotting, the National Institutes of Health has funded a multicenter safety study ("SELENA") to prove that estrogen replacement therapy has no adverse effect on disease activity. This study is ongoing at centers in Baltimore, Los Angeles, and New York. Eligible lupus patients are urged to participate.

Osteoporosis

It is essential that all post-menopausal women with SLE be screened for osteoporosis. All middle-aged men with lupus who have been exposed to prednisone should be screened as well. Screening is currently done with DEXA scans, a nuclear medicine test that gives the patient and the physician a measure of how much bone loss has occurred.

All women who do not have a history of calcium kidney stones should take supplemental calcium, and most will benefit from supplemental vitamin D as well. Healthy habits, such as exercising regularly and not smoking, are helpful in preserving bone density. Two pharmacologic treatments are available for those patients who have moderate to severe osteoporosis. The first treatment is the bisphosphonate group of drugs, which currently includes etidronate, which is given for two weeks on a quarterly basis, and alendronate, which is taken on a daily basis. The second drug that helps to prevent resorption of bone is calcitonin. Calcitonin is now available as a nasal spray, which is well tolerated.

Regardless of whether an elderly patient developed lupus at a young age or after the age of fifty, the challenges to the physician are to manage lupus effectively, while minimizing the side effects of medication. The challenge to the patient is to adopt and maintain good health behaviors—it is never too late!

13

Hormones and Systemic Lupus Erythematosus

by Robert G. Lahita, M.D., Ph.D.

Sex hormones play a very important role in lupus. Most patients realize this importance for several reasons. First, lupus develops most often during the childbearing years, and less commonly before puberty and after menopause. Second, lupus is nine times more common in women than in men. Research indicates that female hormones, called estrogens, may render the immune system more active. In patients with lupus, this changes the overall cell types in the disease, the amount of antibody made, and the patient's symptoms. Some women report that their lupus is most active before their periods begin or that they feel worse when they are pregnant. All of this indicates that sex hormones, which change in amount daily and account for the normal ovulation cycle, play a role in lupus and directly influence its activity.

THE PITUITARY GLAND

When we look at the hormones that affect lupus, we must start with the glands that produce them. The pituitary gland, sometimes called the conductor of the endocrine (glandular) orchestra, sits at the base of the skull. The pituitary is responsible for all of the hormone shifts that take place within the body of both men and women. The pituitary makes chemicals called gonadotropins, which are secreted in a cyclical fashion, permitting women to release eggs from the ovary, menstruate, and produce milk from the breasts. Most scientists now believe that these pituitary agents are cytokines, chemicals that directly affect the immune system.

One such hormone secreted from the pituitary that has been studied extensively is called prolactin. Prolactin is the hormone that causes the breasts to secrete milk. Several scientists from around the world have found that a significant number of their lupus patients have elevated blood levels of prolactin. These scientists have found that the suppression of prolactin with drugs results in clinical improvement for lupus patients. Surprisingly, researchers in this country have not had the same findings. Doubtless, there are other chemicals from the pituitary that have significant effects on immune function. Only now are they coming to light. Chemicals such as growth hormone (a hormone that affects one's rate of growth and the metabolism of some nutrients), luteotrophic hormone (a hormone that influences the secretion of the female hormone progesterone), and follicle-stimulating hormone (a hormone that stimulates the growth of ova in women and sperm in men) are among the group of chemicals that deserve some attention.

THE EFFECTS OF SEX HORMONES ON LUPUS

Sex steroid function in the patient with lupus has been of particular interest, but this part of the endocrine system and its relationship to the immune system has vexed researchers, because the effects that such hormones have on immune function are difficult to sort out. Many scientists have studied the effects of hormones on receptors, those keys that activate cells, in human lymphocytes and have found no difference between those in lupus patients and normal people. Others have studied the levels of sex hormones in lupus patients. Men and women have both male and female hormones in their bodies. However, men have large amounts of male hormones and small amounts of female hormones, and women have large amounts of female hormones and small amounts of male hormones. Researchers thought that perhaps some of the female hormones might be elevated in men and women with lupus. Unfortunately, this has not been the case. What has been found is quite curious. The metabolism of estrogen hormones in people goes toward the very feminizing compounds, whereas the total amount of estrogen compounds never changes. This means that you can metabolize an estrogen to very feminizing compounds without increasing the body's total store of estrogen. Men with lupus are, after all, quite masculine, and, despite numerous attempts to show that they have more estrogen, the data have not shown this.

Some studies of hormone metabolism have indicated that not only has estrogen gone to the very feminizing substances, but also that male hormones called androgens have been very low in women with lupus. This is not found in men. The data indicate that replacement of androgen in women with lupus might serve to weaken the disease, much as it does in animals. This formed the entire basis for the use of the weak androgens like DHEA in the treatment of lupus in women. Since men with lupus have normal levels of male hormones, it is doubtful that replacement of something like a male hormone that is adequate in most men with lupus would do any good. Scientists are currently experimenting with hormones from vegetables and various metabolic byproducts of estrogen, which might help convert the estrogens to the less feminizing variety and increase the male hormone complement to something that will help patients.

Some of the current research in the area of hormones involves an understanding of exactly how and why lupus affects women predominantly. Some new evidence points to the female reproductive system and its immunology. The female and male reproductive systems seem to have their own small population of immune cells that responds to hormones and cytokines in all parts of the body. These secrets began to unravel as physicians noted the high incidence of unusual female reproductive problems that were found in women with lupus.

Lastly, there are major studies proving that hormones can be taken with lupus after menopause and birth control pills might be taken by women with lupus before menopause. It has long been believed that these compounds might not be safe. However, there are no good studies to prove that point. Now the data from a national double-blind study should help clarify these issues.

14

Lupus and Pregnancy

by Michael D. Lockshin, M.D., F.A.C.P.

A woman who has lupus can have a child, though lupus pregnancies are never easy. However, due to early diagnosis, improved prognosis, and changed attitudes, pregnancies in women with systemic lupus erythematosus (SLE), which were once rare, are now commonplace.

Because doctors used to counsel all pregnant women with SLE to undergo therapeutic abortion, the information about lupus and pregnancy available to patients, their families, and their physicians until recently was very limited. Several new studies now provide some answers. This chapter lists the most commonly asked questions of lupus patients considering pregnancy, and answers them citing results of the newest studies.

WILL I BE ABLE TO CONCEIVE?

Fertility (the ability to become pregnant) is normal for most lupus patients. Pregnancy is not likely to occur the first time a patient with lupus has unprotected intercourse, however. It often takes healthy couples up to a year of trying to become pregnant.

Even severe illness usually does not make women sterile, but some of the drugs used to treat lupus—cyclophosphamide (Cytoxan) is the most well known—do reduce fertility. High doses of prednisone often stop a woman's menstrual periods, but patients taking this drug can become pregnant. Thus, unless a woman has been specifically tested and found to be infertile, she should use contraceptives if she wants to avoid pregnancy.

DOES LUPUS FLARE DURING PREGNANCY?

Although textbooks used to say that pregnancy is dangerous for all patients with SLE, since few lupus patients had been allowed to carry their pregnancies, the warning was based on very little solid information. Beginning in the 1980s, several groups of physicians re-examined the issue of lupus and pregnancy, and some things are now clearly understood. First, many lupus patients have no trouble at all with pregnancy. Second, some changes that happen to pregnant women appear to be a flare of lupus but, in fact, are common pregnancy complications not related to lupus. Third, some lupus patients do flare during pregnancy. Whether the number of flares is greater than might be seen if the women were not pregnant is a point about which physicians disagree.

One of the problems of deciding whether flares occur more often in pregnant patients with SLE is that doctors aren't very clear about how often flares usually occur in women who are not pregnant. When doctors compare pregnant lupus patients with lupus patients who are not pregnant, and all factors are considered— age, race, duration of illness, and type and severity of illness—it appears that pregnant women develop flares about as often as do women who are not pregnant. However, when lupus patients' flare rates the year of their pregnancy and the preceding year are compared, studies suggest that flare rates for individual women are higher during pregnancy. Women who have quiet disease at the beginning of pregnancy may be *protected* from flare during pregnancy.

Although it is hard to understand why these apparently contradictory opinions exist, it turns out that such simple factors as when, why, and how a woman is identified for a study explain the different results. Some studies, which enroll women because they have symptoms of lupus during pregnancy, find a high flare rate during pregnancy. This type of study usually comes from a pregnancy clinic in which obstetricians call the rheumatologist conducting the study to tell him or her that a new pregnant lupus patient has been identified. Other studies enroll women who are considering pregnancy. In this case, the rheumatologist usually calls the obstetrician conducting the study to inform him or her that a known patient has become pregnant. This type of study most often finds a low flare rate. In neither case are the patients representative of all lupus patients. The women considering pregnancy have often chosen the time for pregnancy during a period when they are well; and the women with symptoms might not have been identified had they been in complete remission. Unfortunately, there is not yet a clear answer to the question of whether or not the risk of flare is increased by pregnancy.

Although doctors do not agree about the flare risk, they do agree that serious flares are uncommon during pregnancy, that flares in pregnant women can be treated, and that in most cases, pregnancies in those with lupus can continue, even if a flare occurs.

Treatment of the pregnant lupus patient is usually determined by the mother's health and is similar to treatment of patients who are not pregnant. There is no need to treat the mother prophylactically—that is, when she is well—to prevent a flare.

IF I AM PREGNANT, WILL FLARES BE DIFFICULT TO IDENTIFY?

Identifying a flare in a pregnant woman is sometimes difficult because normal effects of pregnancy may look like flares, and because some ways of diagnosing flares are changed by pregnancy. For instance, a decrease in the platelet count or an increase in urine protein, both of which indicate a flare in a lupus patient, can occur in any healthy pregnant woman. Even with special tests, the doctors may not be able to tell whether the findings also indicate that lupus is worsening. On the other hand, a high erythrocyte sedimentation rate (ESR, sed rate), which indicates active SLE, is normal in any pregnancy. Thus, doctors have to use different rules to judge disease activity in a pregnant lupus patient than they do in someone who is not pregnant.

WHAT DRUGS CAN I TAKE DURING PREGNANCY?

It is best, if possible, to take no drugs during pregnancy, but active lupus is worse for the baby than are some commonly used lupus drugs. In no case should the mother's lupus be allowed to worsen during pregnancy simply to reduce the amount of the drugs she takes.

Among drugs used for lupus, aspirin and prednisone are both considered safe to take during pregnancy. There is a debate about the safety of hydroxychloroquine (Plaquenil) and azathioprine (Imuran). No major effects on newborns have been reported, but there has not been much experience with the use of these drugs.

Cyclophosphamide (Cytoxan) causes fetal malformations and miscarriages; it should not be used during pregnancy. Corticosteroid preparations other than prednisone may affect the baby and should not be used. The nonsteroidal anti-inflammatory drugs (NSAIDs) may be safe, but they have not been studied well. I advise not using them.

WILL MY KIDNEY DISEASE WORSEN DURING PREGNANCY?

About one-half of lupus patients have some degree of kidney disease. The worse it is, the more likely it is that there will be problems with pregnancy. The most common problem that occurs in women with kidney disease is a complication of pregnancy called toxemia, or pre-eclampsia. In this condition, the blood pressure rises, protein is excreted in the urine, and fluid collects in the legs and elsewhere. The most effective treatment is for the doctors to deliver the baby as soon as possible, even if the baby will be premature.

Although women with very severe kidney disease—even those who require dialysis—can carry a pregnancy, the risks to both the baby and the mother are very high. As a general rule, if a woman's blood pressure before pregnancy is high enough to need strong medications to keep it normal, or if the kidney function measured by creatinine clearance is more than 25 percent less than normal, pregnancy will likely be a problem.

If a woman with any type of kidney problem gets pregnant, she should be closely monitored throughout her pregnancy by her nephrologist, rheumatologist, and obstetrician.

HOW WILL I BE MONITORED DURING MY PREGNANCY?

There are two types of monitoring, one for the mother and one for the unborn child. For the mother, monthly visits (sometimes more frequent visits) to check for new symptoms and to check urine and blood for signs of lupus activity are often required. The most important factors to watch are the red blood cell count, platelet count, and urine protein. At the beginning of pregnancy, all standard lupus tests are conducted, and antiphospholipid antibody and anti-Ro/SSA and anti-La/SSB antibody levels are determined in order to ensure that the mother is healthy, and so doctors can watch for any changes during the pregnancy.

The fetus is usually checked with an ultrasound test at the beginning of pregnancy, and its growth is monitored by either palpation (feeling the abdomen to determine how big the uterus has become) or by repeated ultrasound tests. In women with anti-Ro/SSA and anti-La/SSB antibodies, an ultrasound test or a fetal electrocardiogram (done from outside the mother's abdomen) may also be used to examine for normality of the heart beat. At approximately twenty-five weeks (six months), especially in women with antiphospholipid antibody or with active SLE, a series of tests for the baby's general health begin. None of these tests are invasive, nor are they painful or dangerous to the mother or the baby. Depending on the situation, they might be done one time only, or they might be done weekly or daily.

SLE itself does not mandate the need for an amniocentesis to be performed (taking a small amount of amniotic fluid through a needle to determine the health of the baby) but amniocentesis might be done for other reasons. If the mother is over the age of thiry-five, for example, an amniocentesis may be performed. Late in pregnancy, if early delivery is likely, amniocentesis might be done to determine if the baby's lungs have matured.

ARE THERE ANY RISKS TO THE BABY?

There are several risks involved in having a baby when you have lupus, but if the disease is closely monitored during the pregnancy, it is quite likely that your baby will be born healthy. There are no specific genetic risks for the child of a woman with SLE. The frequency of Down's syndrome or other malformations is not higher than in the general population. The major risk to the baby is that it will die before it is born (miscarriage). This risk occurs primarily in mothers whose blood contains antiphospholipid antibody.

There are several specific concerns that prospective mothers may have about the effects of their lupus on their unborn child.

Will My Baby Be Born Prematurely?

Premature birth is a risk when the mother has antiphospholipid antibody, when she is very ill, or when the mother develops toxemia. Premature babies have a higher risk of brain damage than do babies born at term. Generally, babies born weighing more than 3 pounds 5 ounces have few problems, though babies weighing less than 2 pounds 3 ounces are at high risk. However, I have seen babies born at 1 pound 7 ounces and grow to be perfectly normal. Different clinics report different rates of prematurity. Although prematurity rates as high as 50 percent have been reported, most babies weigh more than 3 pounds 5 ounces at birth and do well.

Will My Lupus Affect My Baby's Intellectual Development?

In the first few months of life, the growth and development of babies born to mothers with SLE seem normal, taking into account that many of them have been born prematurely. There is very little information available about babies beyond the tod-dler stage. We have re-examined children between five and eight years old. By and large they are doing well in school—some extremely well—and they look like any average group of children of this age. Early fears that there would be a high fre-quency of brain injury in children born to mothers with lupus do not appear to be justified, but questions about a high frequency of mild reading disabilities are not yet fully answered.

What Is Neonatal Lupus, and Will My Child Be More Likely to Have It?

Approximately one-third of women with SLE have anti-Ro/SSA and/or anti-La/SSB antibodies. The children of these women can develop a condition known as neonatal lupus.

Neonatal lupus is not SLE and does not turn into SLE. It consists mostly of a rash, often brought about by sun exposure, that lasts a few weeks and then disap-pears leaving no trace. Babies sometimes have abnormalities of their blood counts that usually need no treatment, since the counts return to normal spontaneously.

A rare manifestation of neonatal lupus, called heart block, is more serious. In this condition, the baby develops a very slow heart beat and sometimes needs a pacemaker after birth. This problem can usually be identified by fetal electrocar-diograms or echocardiograms performed between the eighteenth and twenty-fifth weeks of pregnancy. But even if identified, the slow heart beat cannot be readily treated before birth. The baby's general health is monitored throughout the rest of the pregnancy, and he or she generally will be delivered if in trouble. Fewer than one percent of all lupus patients, and fewer than 3 percent of all women with anti-bodies to both Ro/SSA and La/SSB antigens, deliver babies with this problem. Babies of mothers who have antibodies to neither or to only one of the antigens are not at risk for this heart problem.

Will My Baby Develop Lupus?

The risk that the baby of a mother with lupus will develop lupus is the same as the risk that the mother's brothers or sisters or parents will develop lupus. Most doc-tors think this risk is about one percent. Since the neonatal lupus syndrome has been only recently identified, follow-up studies of children who have had neonatal lupus is quite sparse, but there have been no specific early warnings that these chil-dren are any more susceptible to develop adult lupus than are children who have not had neonatal lupus.

WHAT IS ANTIPHOSPHOLIPID ANTIBODY, AND HOW DOES IT AFFECT PREGNANCY?

Antiphospholipid antibodies attack phospholipids, which are components of cell membranes. There are several different types of antiphospholipid antibodies, including the anticardiolipin antibody and the lupus anticoagulant. Anticardiolipin antibody was the first antiphospholipid antibody described, so the term was once used to describe all antiphospholipid antibodies; however, antibodies can be found against many other phospholipids, so the general term antiphospholipid antibody is now preferred. Some lupus patients have an abnormality in a common blood clotting test that is often used before surgery, but their coagulation (blood clotting) is normal. This abnormality is due to an antiphospholipid antibody called the lupus anticoagulant. Pregnant patients who have the antiphospholipid antibody—about one-third of lupus patients—may miscarry between the fourth and seventh month. The miscarriages seem to be caused by excessive blood clotting in the placenta. Many patients who have antiphospholipid antibodies do not actually have lupus as we now diagnose it. Doctors use the term primary antiphospholipid antibody syndrome (PAPS) to describe those patients who have the antibody but do not have SLE. Antiphospholipid antibodies are not related to any other autoantibody (antibodies against components of one's own body) that lupus patients have.

Not all pregnant patients with antiphospholipid antibody miscarry. In general, a woman who has previously been able to carry a pregnancy to term will carry future pregnancies to term without treatment. Women who have lost at least two pregnancies are those for whom treatment is recommended. There is controversy about whether women who are pregnant for the first time or who have lost only one pregnancy should be treated.

Most doctors now treat pregnant women who have had prior unsuccessful pregnancies with aspirin and/or heparin to prevent blood clotting in the placenta. High-dose prednisone therapy (more than 30 mg per day) was also used previously, but new data indicate that the risk to the mother with this therapy may outweigh the benefits. Some doctors prescribe low doses of prednisone, and there are a variety of experimental types of therapy. Large-scale studies now being planned will soon provide more definitive answers regarding the best treatment.

IF MY MATE HAS LUPUS WILL IT AFFECT THE BABY?

There have been no large-scale studies of children of fathers with lupus, but most studies of men with lupus have noted that they are normally fertile, and that their babies have been normal.

IF I GET PREGNANT, WILL I HAVE TO HAVE A CESAREAN SECTION TO DELIVER?

Lupus patients do not universally have to deliver by cesarean section. The need to do this is dictated by specific obstetrical considerations that involve either the baby's or the mother's health at the time of delivery. However, since in many cases the mother or the child is ill, lupus patients are more likely to need a cesarean section for delivery than are women who do not have lupus.

CAN I BREAST-FEED MY BABY?

There is very little direct information available about lupus and breast-feeding. Many mothers have done so with no apparent harm to themselves or to their infants. It is, however, difficult to breast-feed premature infants, and women taking prednisone often do not produce breast milk. Many drugs taken by the mother pass through the breast milk to the baby, so a mother taking drugs should talk to her doctor before starting breast-feeding.

CAN A WOMAN WITH LUPUS TAKE BIRTH CONTROL PILLS?

Several medical articles published in the late 1970s and early 1980s suggested that birth control pills cause lupus to flare; thus most physicians told their patients not to take oral contraceptives. It is now believed that the extreme caution of the 1970s was excessive, though no new studies have been done. But many lupus patients do take birth control pills now with no apparent effects. Nonetheless, extreme caution with birth control pills is recommended. Since one of the possible complications of anyone's use of birth control pills is increased blood clotting that leads to phlebitis and stroke—similar to what occurs in antiphospholipid antibody syndrome—women with the antiphospholipid antibody should not take oral contraceptives.

Condoms, diaphragms, most spermicidal jellies, and intrauterine devices are generally safe for lupus patients. There is no information about the effect of the new implantable contraceptive (Norplant) on lupus patients.

IS IT DANGEROUS FOR A WOMAN WITH LUPUS TO HAVE AN ABORTION?

There are no special risks for termination of pregnancy in women with SLE, other than those associated with medical procedure. There is no experience with the "morning-after" pill (RU-486) in women with lupus.

WHAT RECOURSES DO I HAVE IF I WANT TO HAVE CHILDREN BUT AM UNABLE?

Generally, lupus does not affect one's fertility, though some drugs used to treat the disease may reduce one's fertility. For infertile women who are having difficulties getting pregnant, a variety of techniques are available to help. In some women, hormones are given to induce eggs to develop and be released. In others, extra hormones are given early in pregnancy. Hormone treatment is especially common in GIFT and ZIFT (Gamete or Zygote-Intra-Fallopian Tube Transplant) pregnancies in which an egg is fertilized outside the body and then placed into the womb. The lupus patient who does not produce eggs can be artificially inseminated with another woman's egg fertilized by her husband's sperm.

If a lupus patient can produce eggs but is too ill to support a pregnancy, she can consider a surrogate pregnancy, in which her fertilized egg is implanted into the womb of another woman (a surrogate), who will carry the baby to term and deliver it. There are no systematic studies of such pregnancies in women with lupus, but carefully selected patients have undergone these procedures successfully. Adoption is another option for those having problems conceiving. However, several, even those in full remission for more than a decade, have often faced severe, insensitive, and cruel opposition from adoption agencies.

All physicians who see lupus patients know several who have normal grown children. There has never been a systematic follow-up of a large number of children of lupus mothers, though alarms have been raised from time to time about their growth and intellectual development. In our own studies we are now looking at the now school-aged children born of lupus mothers. Preliminary results suggest that when matched for birth weight they look pretty much like other children, and they are doing well in school. They do not appear to have unusual health problems. From past information we know that their risk of developing lupus themselves is quite low. Prospective parents should consider how the baby will be cared for if the mother is ill.

Pregnancy does not cure lupus. The new mother, or the family considering pregnancy, should keep in mind that the mother has an important illness, that this illness is unlikely to go away, and that there may be periods during which the mother cannot care for the growing child. Exhaustion is always a threat to the mother, but a newborn, hungry in the middle of the night, or a two-year-old, full of energy, will not understand this. Nor will a child understand if Mom has to stay in bed or has to go to the hospital. The family support systems have to be very strong. In most cases, the father will have to provide immediate back-up. Some families are lucky enough to have in-laws available, and some families are lucky enough to be able to hire help. Each family should think of the potential problems before the baby arrives and have solutions available to them. Fathers should capitalize on any family-leave policies that may be available at their places of employment and should fully participate in raising the child. Lupus pregnancies are difficult, but with support and cooperation, they can be extremely rewarding.

PART FOUR

Manisfestations of Lupus

15

How Can One Classify Lupus?

by Henrietta Aladjem
in Conversation With Chester Alper, M.D.

Over a cup of coffee, I asked Dr. Chester Alper, who was one of my doctors when I was first diagnosed with lupus, how lupus is classified. Dr. Alper responded that no single system of classification is accepted and used by all physicians. In some cases, lupus can be classified by organ of involvement. After a brief pause, he said, "It would be hard to imagine a disease with more varied clinical manifestations and, therefore, signs and symptoms and multiple organ involvement than lupus. As we all know, any single patient may have only mild disease, with few symptoms or signs or many different symptoms and signs, all at once, or spread out over many years. At any given moment, a group of patients in relapse might have totally different signs and symptoms and nothing in common but the diagnosis of lupus. Since virtually every organ and organ system of the body may be affected in lupus patients, it is clearly unsatisfactory to call lupus a skin disease, or a heart disease, or a lung disease, or a blood disease, even though it is all of these and more."

Dr. Alper continued, "Classifications may also vary with the viewpoint and background of the medical scientists studying a specific aspect of the disease. The result is not unlike the description of the elephant as reported by the blind man. For some years, lupus was called a 'connective tissue' disease because biopsy sections or many organs from patients with systemic lupus showed abnormal stained microscopic appearance of the supporting tissue present throughout the body. Later, this rubric was changed to 'collagen vascular.' Collagen is the primary component of connective tissues, and the word 'vascular' was added to stress involvement of blood vessels. This classification is in current use. Immunologists, on the other hand, were initially struck by the presence of apparent autoantibodies directed against normal body constituents, and called lupus an autoimmune disorder. More recently, it has become clear that the nature of the antigen may be secondary, but that major damage to tissue in lupus may be mediated by antigen-antibody complexes irrespective of the nature of the specific antigen. Therefore, lupus is further referred to as an immune-complex disorder."

I told Dr. Alper that even though lupus patients can have different signs and symptoms and nothing in common but the diagnosis of lupus, the majority of patients share an incredible exhaustion that often defies explanation. "Such a fatigue," I said, "engulfs the spirit and the body . . . At thirty, sometimes you feel like eighty. With pain, you hurt, but you feel alive . . . With the lupus fatigue, you have this morbid sense as if your body is beginning to die."

I had many more questions for Dr. Alper, but he suggested we talk about it over another cup of coffee.

I am presenting a few aspects of the lupus syndrome, as described by several knowledgeable medical investigators and clinicians.

16

Lupus and the Lung

by Daniel J. Wallace, M.D., F.A.C.P.

Normally functioning lungs effortlessly exchange oxygen for carbon dioxide. In systemic lupus, a variety of disease processes can interfere with this mechanism producing shortness of breath, chest pain, rapid breathing, fever, or cough. How does lupus do this? In the next few pages, I will investigate some of the lung disorders that can occur as a result of lupus.

PLEURISY

The lining of the lung—called the pleura—is like a cellophane or "gift wrap" around the organ, but is not part of the lung itself. Inflammation of this lining occurs in most patients with systemic lupus erythematosus (SLE) and leads to pain upon taking a deep breath. Pleurisy responds to high doses of nonsteroidal anti-inflammatory agents, antimalarials, and short courses of steroids. Atrophy of the diaphragm—the muscle that expands the lungs when we breathe—may be caused by chronic pleural scarring. This atrophy is called shrinking lung syndrome, and patients complain of inability to take a deep breath and decreased stamina and endurance.

ACUTE LUPUS PNEUMONITIS

Acute lupus pneumonitis occurs when lung tissue—called interstitium—becomes inflamed by a type of white blood cell known as a granulocyte. To a doctor, this may look just like acute pneumonia or bronchitis, but responds only to high doses of steroids, not antibiotics.

INTERSTITIAL LUNG DISEASE

Interstitial lung disease is a chronic, slowly evolving inflammatory process involving white blood cells known as lymphocytes. Interstitial lung disease induces mild shortness of breath and responds to steroids and immunosuppressive regimens. It is also associated with such overlapping immune conditions as Sjögren's syndrome, scleroderma, or rheumatic arthritis.

PULMONARY EMBOLISM

A pulmonary embolism is the sudden blocking of an artery of a lung, usually by a blood clot. This condition occurs more often in lupus patients who have a lupus anticoagulant or antiphospholipid antibodies. Patients develop sudden onset of chest pain and shortness of breath. They may also experience coughing, blood-streaked sputum, and fever. Hospitalization with intravenous anticoagulation is the treatment of choice followed by oral blood thinners.

PULMONARY HEMORRHAGE

Pulmonary hemorrhage is a condition associated with very active disease. The major symptom is the coughing up of blood. Seen in 3 percent of lupus patients, this serious complication requires aggressive anti-inflammatory management.

PULMONARY HYPERTENSION

Pulmonary hypertension, high blood pressure in the vessels of the lungs, is another serious, often lethal condition. It is characterized by shortness of breath. If left untreated, pulmonary hypertension can cause damage to the blood vessels, lower oxygen levels in the blood, and ultimately cause heart failure. Two-dimensional echocardiography or ultrasound of the heart are used to confirm the diagnosis. If medication fails to control the problem, some patients may need a lung transplant.

BRONCHITIS SICCA

Bronchitis sicca, or dry lungs, is part of Sjögren's syndrome, a condition that often accompanies lupus. Manifested by dry eyes, dry mouth, and arthritis, Sjögren's syndrome is seen in 20 percent of lupus patients. Patients have a dry, hacking, non-productive cough. Managed by humidification regimens such as chicken soup, steam showers, vaporizers, room humidifiers, or drugs (e.g., Humabid), this is a chronic and frustrating process that is rarely serious.

OTHER LUNG PROBLEMS

Occasionally, medications used to treat lupus, such as aspirin, nonsteroidal anti-inflammatory drugs, or methotrexate, can induce asthma or shortness of breath. Lupus patients are also at high risk of lung infection, and the presence of fever usually warrants treatment for an infection. Also, some chest pain and discomfort may have other causes, such as heart problems, esophageal spasm, gastritis, ulcer, or arthritis of the chest wall (costochondritis).

When a patient presents with pulmonary-related symptoms, doctors usually take a history, ask about possible environmental or occupational exposures, and listen to the chest for a signal of asthma, pneumonia, or bronchitis. Conducting a panel of blood tests, a complete blood count, and a chest x-ray is the usual starting point. If necessary, additional testing, such as a CT scan, blood gas test, pulmonary function testing, electrocardiogram, upper GI series, or chest ultrasound, may be ordered.

As can be seen, chest complaints can result from a variety of sources and range from those that are easily treatable to serious disorders. Doctors need to take all chest complaints seriously, and can usually make a correct diagnosis rather quickly with a focused examination.

17

Osteonecrosis, Avascular Necrosis, Aseptic Necrosis, Osteoporosis, and Total Hip Replacement

by Michael D. Lockshin, M.D., F.A.C.P.

Osteonecrosis. Avascular necrosis. Aseptic necrosis. Osteoporosis. Total hip replacement. These are terms that confuse lupus patients. Unfortunately, they represent medical issues (sometimes legal issues) that receive an inappropriately small amount of attention when doctors talk to patients.

"'An inappropriately small amount of attention?' What do you mean?" you may ask. I say this because these skeletal problems are important long-term issues in the lives of lupus patients, and because they are primarily complications of corticosteroid therapy, they force us to reevaluate what doctors say about side effects of treatment. Skeletal complications also make us think about what patients really want to know and when.

First, what do the terms mean?

OSTEONECROSIS

Osteonecrosis, avascular necrosis, and aseptic necrosis are synonyms. Osteonecrosis means death of bone tissue ("osteo-" means bone, "-necrosis" means tissue death), avascular necrosis ("a-" means without, "vascular" means blood vessel) refers to the fact that bone dies when it loses its blood supply. Aseptic necrosis ("a-" means without, "-septic" means infection) distinguishes the osteonecrosis that happens to lupus patients from that caused by infection.

In osteonecrosis, a small section of bone dies. It happens most often in the ball of the ball-and-socket hip joint. The bone becomes soft and unable to bear weight, and it collapses. When that happens, the hip becomes very painful and hard to move. There are some treatments that can shore up the ball before it collapses, but usually patients with osteonecrosis of the hip need a joint replacement. Osteonecrosis can occur in other areas of the body. In some places, like the shoulder, it is debilitating but can be repaired. Osteonecrosis in other parts of the body may cause no symptoms. Osteonecrosis can occur in people who do not have lupus, often due to corticosteroid therapy, and it can occur in lupus patients who have never been treated. The combination of lupus and high-dose (60 milligrams or more of prednisone per day for several weeks) corticosteroid therapy is particularly hard on bones. Ten to 20 percent of lupus patients who have been thus treated will develop osteonecrosis. Often the osteonecrosis does not become apparent until two to five years after the high-dose corticosteroid treatment period is over.

OSTEOPOROSIS

Osteoporosis is a different problem. "-Porosis" means pores or holes, so osteoporosis refers to thinning of bone throughout the body. In the spinal column, osteoporosis leads to back pain and a bent back, both due to the collapse of weakened vertebrae. In the hip, osteoporosis leads to fracture. Women's bones are made strong by estrogen; after menopause, when estrogen production decreases, women's bones thin. Corticosteroid therapy may cause or exacerbate bone thinning in both sexes. Corticosteroid-associated osteoporosis takes years to develop and, once present, may not reverse. Prevention of postmenopausal osteoporosis is the reason women are advised to take calcium at all ages and estrogen after menopause. There are many questions about the possible negative effects of supplemental estrogen in lupus patients, so women with lupus are advised against undergoing estrogen therapy. Many of these women are taking corticosteroids, so their bones are in double jeopardy. A national study now underway, funded by the National Institutes of Health (NIH), is looking at whether women with lupus can safely use estrogen. Many doctors think they can.

HIP REPLACEMENT

Total hip replacement is the surgical procedure most often used to treat osteonecrosis, and it is often performed when a hip fractures. The ball and neck of the hip bone and usually the socket part of the joint are replaced with a metal and plastic prosthesis. After hip replacement, patients can be free of pain with normal use of the joint. (Horseback riding and skiing are *not* advised!) A hip replacement is not always permanent; it may deteriorate and need to be replaced again. With today's materials and surgical techniques, hip replacements that last more than ten years are common.

The skeletal complications discussed above are, for the most part, complications of corticosteroid therapy. The higher the corticosteroid dose, the longer treatment period, the more likely osteonecrosis or osteoporosis will occur. What is not often discussed is how much, and when, should the doctor tell the patient about the skeletal toxicity of corticosteroid therapy?

Generally, doctors do inform the patient of potential side effects of drugs that they prescribe. The problem occurs when a patient has the potential to develop kidney failure, brain damage, life-threatening hemorrhaging, or some other catastrophe. These are critical problems, and while there is a treatment to prevent such occurrences, telling the patient about frightening side effects of the drug may scare him or her out of using the therapy. In these cases, doctors are often selective about what they tell the patient. Certainly, however, the patient should be involved in this decision-making process, and should be fully aware of all of the potential side effects of any treatment. This issue must be addressed by physicians and patients alike.

18

Behavior in Lupus Mice: A Lesson for Human C.N.S. Lupus

by Judah A. Denburg, M.D., F.R.C.P.

After I gave a lecture in Toronto and was on the same panel with Dr. Judah A. Denburg, a Professor of Medicine, McMaster University, I asked him to write an article for Lupus Letter *and for* The Challenges of Lupus *about his studying of the involvement of the nervous system of patients with lupus. This is what he wrote.*

For many years, a reasearch group at McMaster University, including Susan A. Denburg, Ph.D., professor, Department of Psychiatry; Boris Sakic, Ph.D., assistant professor, Department of Psychiatry; Henry Szechtman, Ph.D., professor, Department of Biomedical Sciences; and me, has been studying the involvement of the nervous system in patients with lupus. By now, it is well established, not only in our laboratory but in several others, that many patients with lupus have problems in both cognitive (i.e., related to thinking skills) and affective (i.e., having to do with emotional issues) areas. For example, patients with lupus have difficulties remembering things they have studied or learned, coming up with the right word at the appropriate time, concentrating or attending to details, or figuring out directions. In addition, patients with lupus can have mood swings, be irritable, have difficulties relating to their spouses, or experience extreme emotional and mental fatigue, often without any obvious flare-ups of lupus.

We have shown that these difficulties in the cognitive and affective areas are related to the presence of certain autoantibodies found in the blood or cerebrospinal fluid that are directed against the nervous system. However, we have not been able to prove that these autoantibodies, or for that matter, any other factors, actually *directly* cause the cognitive and affective problems in lupus patients. The difficulty has been mainly in studying the brain, since it is not as easy to look inside the brain tissue as it is, for example, to study the kidney by performing a biopsy and examining the types of kidney inflammation in lupus. Therefore, it has become important in recent years to turn our attention to animals with lupus and see whether or not they develop nervous system problems similar to humans with lupus, so that we can understand the mechanism and develop strategies in a more reasonable fashion.

ANIMAL MODELS OF LUPUS

There are several different animal species that develop lupus; principal among these are mice, which can develop many of the features of lupus spontaneously during the course of a life span. In mice, there are several different strains (subtypes within a given species) that develop lupus or lupuslike disease: One is called the NZB/W mouse, which develops lupus rather slowly over more than a year. This lupus is characterized predominantly by involvement of the blood and kidneys, with the presence of many typical autoantibodies, such as anti-DNA antibodies and ANA (antinuclear antibodies). Affected mice are also known to have some learning difficulties, especially in the tasks that require them to use their memories to avoid something unpleasant, such as an electric shock. However, the NZB/W mice take months to develop full-blown lupus.

Another animal model is the MRL mouse, which develops lupus quite rapidly between the ages of 3 weeks and 16 weeks of age, with arthritis, hemolytic anemia, kidney abnormalities, salivary gland enlargement, as occurs in Sjögren's syndrome, and many typical autoantibodies in the blood. The disease is rapidly progressive in these animals and ends with a life-threatening illness involving the lymph nodes that resembles lymphoma.

Clearly, neither of these lupus models (nor other mouse lupus models) is identical to humans with SLE. This is because human lupus is a mixture of many factors, including genetic and environmental ones. However, in animal models, all the mice of a given strain are almost identical. So, lupus mice can give us a picture of what can happen when lupus is "condensed" into one uniform disease: They fulfill almost all the criteria for lupus rather than only several. We can also predict a lot of different abnormalities in human lupus from animal models and learn a great deal about their mechanisms and treatment. This has been done for kidney involvement and perhaps is very relevant to nervous system involvement as well.

Behavioral Problems in MRL Mice

We undertook several studies over the last six years to investigate whether or not MRL mice have behavioral problems resembling or related to human CNS lupus. We were extremely surprised to find that from the age of 3 to 4 weeks, at a time when autoantibodies are just forming, but the disease itself has not yet developed fully, these mice are very different in their behaviors compared with their littermates who do not have lupus but otherwise are almost genetically identical. The typical abnormalities in behavior seen in these mice are a hesitancy to explore new environments or touch or sniff new objects and a decrease in normal activity. Moreover, these mice cannot learn as well the spatial location of an escape platform in a water maze. In fact, these animals give up quickly and float in a helpless fashion if they cannot escape. These behaviors are seen in mice when they suffer repeated unavoidable stress. This learned helplessness can usually be reversed by antidepressant drugs, meaning that it may represent a form of depression.

The MRL mice also develop abnormalities in their thinking skills. It takes them longer to learn where the platform was moved to than it does for their "normal" littermates, and several other indicators suggest that they cannot remember things normally. Thus, the animals have both an affective and a cognitive abnormality that genetically very similar mice do not have. What intrigued us was the question of what could cause this array of abnormalities? How could it be present so early in the course of disease? Why did this continue to get relatively worse with age?

The Brain in MRL Mice

To answer some of the questions that arose, we have to know a little more about the abnormalities in the brain and immune system in lupus mice in general. In several studies it has been found that the brains of lupus MRL mice have accumulations of white blood cells, indicating inflammation. It looks as if an immune response is occurring in the MRL mouse brain, since some of the brain cells that normally keep the brain properly functioning are "activated," much like they are in the earliest phase of inflammation in, for example, the joints. Moreover, in some other strains of mice and in MRL mice, there are structural abnormalities of the brain, which may be related to the behavioral problems. And finally, there are changes in neurotransmitters, communicating molecules that allow the brain's activity to proceed normally; or in cytokines, immune system molecules that are found in normal human and mouse brains. Cytokines influence responses to stress and the body's ability to make corticosteroids. The corticosteroid hormonal system is called the hypothalamic-pituitary-adrenal (HPA) axis, which is of vital importance in regulating normal behavior, appetite, temperature, fatigue and response to stress; in MRL as well as other lupus mice, there appear to be abnormalities in the HPA axis and cytokines that may significantly affect behavior.

Links Between the Brain and Behavior in MRL Mice

How can we link the brain abnormalities with the abnormal behaviors we have observed in MRL mice? One way is to recreate the same abnormal situation of MRL mice in the brains of normal mice and see if the behaviors that are seen in MRL mice are also found in these altered normal mice. We had observed an increased level of cytokine interleukin-6 (IL-6) in MRL mice, so we decided to increase the level of IL-6 in normal mice or in the MRL control mice that do not normally develop behavioral abnormalities. What we found was astonishing: The higher the IL-6 level in normal mice, the more likely they were to develop depressive behaviors. Of particular interest was the development of learned helplessness, as well as a lack of interest in drinking a sweet solution, which is also a marker of depressive behavior. Thus, what spontaneously occurs in our MRL lupus mice could be recreated in normal mice simply by increasing, temporarily, the IL-6 levels in the blood and cerebrospinal fluid. Since IL-6 is elevated in lots of inflammatory reactions, we have a clue now that one of the important causes of some abnormal behaviors in MRL mice is an increased IL-6 level.

Treatment of MRL Behavioral Abnormalities

We also gave the MRL lupus mice cyclophosphamide, an immunosuppressive drug used in human lupus to control disease of the kidneys. When we gave this medication in doses that could control lupus in these mice, but at a point in time much before lupus really was all over the body, we could reverse many of the depressivelike behaviors, such as the excessive floating in the water maze and the hesitancy to touch new objects. Cyclophosphamide, a drug that suppresses autoimmune responses, could reverse abnormal behavior. Also, the animals whose behavior became normal after cyclophosphamide were the ones in whom both the inflammation (white blood cells in the brain) disappeared and the IL-6 levels fell to normal. This suggested very strongly that an excessively active immune system was the reason for the behavioral abnormalities.

We have also been exploring the effects of antidepressant drugs on the abnormal behaviors in lupus mice, since some of these may mimic human SLE-related depression, an important clinical issue. While we do not have all the results to date, some of our findings suggest that certain antidepressants may be more effective than others in lupus mice; in fact, some of the MRL lupus mice are very sensitive to low doses of typical antidepressants and may actually get worse with them if we are not too careful. Thus, the changes in the brain may be quite complex and require new kinds of medications that target both the immune and nervous systems simultaneously.

Future Directions

Knowing that the brain is inflamed in lupus and that infiltration by cells and effects of cytokines can lead to both neurologic and psychiatric (i.e., behavioral) abnormalities, we are gaining confidence in using the animal model to plan the future of therapy for CNS lupus. The literature on the brain in human lupus is very meager, since autopsy findings are scarce and controlled studies are virtually nonexistent. Using animal models to construct new approaches to controlling cytokine responses, altering inflammation-causing genes, and manipulating the immune response via changes in stress and environment, may all help us understand the complex interaction between the immune and nervous systems in autoimmune disease. What is beginning to emerge is the knowledge that autoimmunity can directly affect the brain, and that the brain in autoimmune animals, and possibly in people with SLE, is "turned on" in such a way as to lead to behavioral and other nervous system abnormalities. Thus, the key to changing and reversing cognitive and affective problems in patients with lupus is probably the same key that is required to turn off the autoimmune response in the organism as a whole.

19

Cardiac Manifestations of Systemic Lupus Erythematosus

by Peter H. Schur, M.D.

*D*r. *Peter H. Schur and I have worked as a team for more than twenty years, and I have always regarded him as not only my mentor, but as a friend. Since my own physician, Dr. Frank Gardner, moved to Texas, Dr. Schur has also taken over my medical care.*

Recently, I developed a mild heart condition, and it came to my attention that heart problems are common in lupus patients. I asked Dr. Schur to write something about the cardiac manifestations of lupus for this book. He promptly sent me a paper he had written on the subject, and it is printed here for you to read.

Cardiac disease is common among patients with systemic lupus erythematosus (SLE). Pericardial, myocardial, valvular, and coronary artery involvement can occur. Several studies have also described associations of valvular disease with antiphospholipid antibodies. The incidence of these problems can be summarized as follows:

- Cardiac abnormalities—up to 55 percent.[1]

- Valvular disease, most often mitral regurgitation and usually hemodynamically insignificant—up to 50 percent.[2]

- Pericardial disease, usually a clinically silent effusion—up to 48 percent.[1]

- Myocardial dysfunction—up to 78 percent.[2]

- Coronary artery disease—about 2 to 3 percent.[1]

VALVULAR DISEASE

Systolic murmurs (those that occur during the contraction of the heart) have been noted in 16 to 44 percent of all lupus patients.[1] Structural valvular disease is the most common cause,[2–6] but anemia, fever, tachycardia (fast heartbeat), and cardiomegaly (enlarged heart) can induce functional murmurs. Diastolic murmurs (those that occur during relaxation of the heartbeat) have been noted in 1 to 3 percent of patients.[1] They often reflect aortic insufficiency, which occasionally requires valve replacement.

Some studies suggest an association between valvular disease and antiphospho-lipid antibodies.[2,7–9] In one report, for example, 78 percent of patients with high levels of antiphospholipid antibodies had at least one cardiac abnormality.[9] Patients with mild pulmonary hypertension, a less common complication of lupus, are also more likely to have antiphospholipid antibodies.[9] However, other reports have not confirmed the suspected relationship between antiphospholipid antibodies and cardiac disease.[2,10,11]

Mitral valve involvement is most common; a mild to moderate regurgitant murmur (a murmur due to valve leakage) may be heard but most patients remain asymptomatic.[3,8,10] Mitral valve prolapse appears to occur with increased frequency in lupus, occurring in 25 percent of lupus patients in another study versus 9 percent of controls.[10]

A recent report used transesophageal echocardiography to determine the frequency, clinical course, and complications of valvular disease in sixty-nine patients with SLE, most of whom underwent a second study a mean of twenty-nine months later.[4] The following findings were noted:

- Thickening of the leaflets (the cusps of the valves) was the most common, occurring in 51 and 52 percent of patients at the two study times. This lesion is due to initial valvulitis (inflammation of the valves) followed by healing with fibrosis and thickening.

- Valvular vegetations were present in 43 and 34 percent of patients.

- Valvular regurgitation was noted in 28 percent at both time periods.

- Valvular stenosis (constriction of the valves), which was not progressive, was found in 4 and 3 percent.

- The manifestations of valvular disease frequently changed: some revolved, others appeared for the first time, and some changed their appearance.

- Neither the presence nor changes in valvular disease were temporally related to disease activity, therapy, or the duration of SLE.

- Perhaps most importantly, there was an appreciable incidence of serious complications in the patients with valvular disease. After a mean follow-up of almost five years, the combined incidence of stroke, peripheral embolism, heart failure, infective endocarditis, and death was 22 percent versus 15 percent in the thirteen patients without valvular disease. The incidence of stroke in patients with valvular disease was 13 percent.

If these data were broadly applicable, then all patients with lupus would require continuing serial echocardiographic monitoring to detect and treat the development of new, potentially serious valvular lesions. However, I personally have not seen the high incidence of complications from valvular disease reported in this study, although we routinely listen to patients' hearts at most visits, followed by the use of echocardiography for the evaluation of significant or changing murmurs or changing cardiac function. The reason for this discrepancy is not known.

Plasma homocysteine levels appear to be another risk factor for stroke in SLE (and in the general population). A prospective study from the Hopkins Lupus

Cohort Study evaluated 337 patients with SLE for a mean duration of 4.8 years.[12] The endpoints were stroke or arterial or venous thrombotic events. After adjustment for established risk factors, an increase of one log unit of plasma homocysteine concentration was an independent risk factor for both stroke and arterial thromboses (relative risk 2.44 and 3.49 respectively).

Libman-Sacks (or verrucous) endocarditis (inflammation of the interior lining of the heart, with the presence of warts) is a common complication of SLE. In one report of seventy-four patients, for example, seven had verrucous lesions detected by transthoracic echocardiography.[3] As noted above, however, 43-percent more are detected when more sensitive transesophageal echocardiography is performed.[4] In addition, Libman-Sacks endocarditis is often associated with antiphospholipid antibodies.[7]

The verrucae (warts) are usually near the edge of the valve and consist of accumulations of immune complexes, mononuclear cells, hematoxylin bodies, and fibrin and platelet thrombi. The mitral, aortic, and tricuspid valves are more often involved.[1] Healing usually leads to fibrosis, scarring, and, in some cases, calcification. If the verrucal lesions are extensive, the healing process can produce deformity of the valve, possibly leading to mitral or aortic regurgitation.

Verrucous endocarditis is typically asymptomatic. However, the verrucae can fragment and produce systemic emboli, and infective endocarditis can develop on already damaged valves.[1,4] Blood cultures and echocardiography should be performed whenever fever and a new murmur are noted in an SLE patient.[2] In addition, one can consider antibiotic prophylaxis for SLE patients undergoing procedures associated with a risk of valvular bacteremia (such as dental care).[13]

PERICARDIAL DISEASE

Pericardial involvement is the second most common echocardiographic lesion in SLE, and is the most frequent cause of symptomatic cardiac disease. Pericardial effusion occurs at some point in over half of patients, and a benign pericarditis may precede the clinical signs of lupus.

Characteristics

Pericardial disease is usually asymptomatic, and is generally diagnosed by echocardiography performed for some other reason, such as suggestive electrocardiographic abnormalities.[14] Symptomatic pericarditis typically presents with positional substernal chest pain with an audible rub on auscultation (listening to the heart). There may also be signs of serositis, such as pleural effusion and ascites, at other sites.

The pericardial fluid is a fibrinous exudate or transudate that may contain antinuclear antibodies, LE cells, low complement levels, and immune complexes similar to those seen in lupus pleural effusions.[15] The glucose concentration is normal and the protein concentration is variable, being low with a transudate and elevated with an exudate. The pericardium may reveal foci of inflammatory lesions with immune complexes. There is usually a predominance of mononuclear cells, but scarring may be the primary finding in healed disease.

Course and Treatment

The course is benign in the large majority of patients with pericardial disease. Symptomatic pericarditis often responds to a nonsteroidal anti-inflammatory drug, especially indomethacin.[1] Patients who do not tolerate or respond to an NSAID can be treated with prednisone (0.5 to 1 mg/kg per day in divided doses). The most serious consequence is the development of purulent (producing pus) pericarditis in the immunosuppressed, debilitated patient.[16] Large effusions, suggestive of tamponade (compression of the heart due to accumulation of fluid in the pericardium), and constrictive pericarditis are rare in SLE.[17]

MYOCARDITIS

Myocarditis is inflammation of the heart. It is an uncommon, often asymptomatic manifestation of SLE with a prevalence of 8 to 25 percent in different studies.[1]

Characteristics

Myocarditis should be suspected if there is resting tachycardia disproportionate to body temperature, electrocardiographic abnormalities (such as ST and T wave—those waves that indicate recovery after a heartbeat—abnormalities), and unexplained cardiomegaly. The cardiomegaly may be associated with symptoms and signs of congestive heart failure, conductive abnormalities, and/or arrhythmias. Echocardiography may reveal abnormalities in both systolic and diastolic function of the left ventricle. Myocarditis has been associated in some cases with antibodies to ribonucleoprotein and extractable nuclear antigen.[18]

Acute myocarditis may accompany other manifestations of acute SLE, particularly pericarditis. Histologic examination reveals infiltration of the myocardium with mononuclear cells. Resolution of the inflammation leads to fibrosis that may be manifested clinically as dilated cardiomyopathy (a disorder in which the ventricles are enlarged but unable to pump enough blood, which can result in heart failure). Myocardial biopsy may be needed to distinguish active myocarditis from fibrosis.[19]

Treatment

Myocarditis should be treated with prednisone (1 mg/kg per day in divided doses), plus usual therapy for congestive heart failure if present. A few patients have been treated with cyclophosphamide or azathioprine.[20,21] Cardiomyopathy is usually resistant to steroids and/or immunosuppressive drugs.

CONDUCTION ABNORMALITIES

Conduction defects, which may represent a sequel of active or past pericarditis and/or myocarditis, have been noted in 34 to 70 percent of patients with SLE.[1] First-degree heart block may be seen and is often transient; in comparison, higher degrees of heart block and arrhythmias (such as atrial fibrillation) are unusual in adults. Autopsy studies have revealed focal inflammatory cell infiltrates or, more often, fibrous scarring of the conduction system. Congenital heart block may be part of the neonatal lupus syndrome. Many mothers of these infants have either SLE or Sjögren's syndrome, antibodies to Ro (SS-A) and/or La (SS-B), and are HLA-DR3 positive.[21] The anti-Ro and anti-La antibodies may induce autoimmune injury that prevents normal development of the conduction fibers.[22] It is therefore recommended that anti-Ro antibody titers be measured early in pregnancy in women with SLE. The resting heart rate may correlate with disease activity. In one report, fourteen of fifteen patients with a resting heart rate above 90 beats/min had active disease.[23]

CORONARY ARTERY DISEASE

Coronary artery disease has been recognized in 2 to 3 percent of patients with SLE,[24-27] and can lead to acute myocardial infarction (heart attack) in young women.[25,26] In some cases, however, thrombi, rather than coronary disease, are responsible for the ischemia.[28]

In our experience and that of others, coronary disease, leading to angina, myocardial infarction, congestive heart failure, and death, is becoming an increasing problem, particularly in the young patients with long-standing SLE maintained on corticosteroids.[25,26,29,30] One author has noted the bimodal character of mortality in SLE: infection due in part to immunosuppression is most common in the early course, while coronary disease is more prominent after two years.[29] In another report, coronary disease (defined as angina, myocardial infarction, or sudden death) occurred in 8.3 percent of 229 patients and was responsible for three of ten deaths.[26]

Pathogenesis

The factors responsible for premature coronary disease are incompletely understood. An increased incidence of risk factors (some nontraditional) for atherosclerosis has been noted. In one study, for example, three or more risk factors were found in 53 percent of a cohort of 229 patients with a mean age of only 38.3 years.[25] These include hypertension, obesity, lipid abnormalities,[31-34] corticosteroids (which can cause or exacerbate hyperlipidemia and obesity),[32] increased plasma homocysteine concentrations,12 chronic nephritis,[35] low serum levels of C3,[36] elevated levels of antibodies to dsDNA,[36] and antiphospholipid antibodies[37,38] (which promote thrombosis). It has also been proposed that autoimmune vascular injury leading to coronary arteritis may predispose patients to atherosclerotic plaque formation[39].

The importance of these factors can be illustrated by the clinical differences that have been noted in patients with coronary disease when compared with those without coronary disease[26]:

- Increased age at diagnosis of SLE (37.1 versus 28.9 years) and at entry into the study (47.1 years versus 34.7 years).

- Longer mean duration of SLE (12.3 versus 8.1 years).

- Longer mean duration of prednisone use (14.3 versus 7.2 years).

- Higher mean plasma cholesterol concentration (271 versus 215 mg/dL [7.0 versus 5.6 mmol/L]) and more frequent occurrence of a cholesterol level above 200 mg/dL (5.2 mmol/L).

- Greater prevalence of hypertension and a history of use of antihypertensive medication.

The specific effect of prednisone and hydroxychloroquine on coronary risk factors was studied in a cohort of 264 patients.[40] The administration of hydroxychloroquine produced a decrease in plasma cholesterol of 8.9 mg/dL (0.23 mmol/L). In contrast, in a regression model corrected for age, weight, and antihypertensive dose, a 10 mg/day increase in prednisone dose led to definable worsening of the following risk factors:

- An increase in serum cholesterol of 7.5 mg/dL (0.19 mmol/L).

- An increase in mean arterial blood pressure of 1.1 mmHg.

- An increase in body weight of 2.5 kg.

Prevention and Treatment

Patients with SLE should be made aware of the importance of risk factor reduction. In one study, for example, only 17 percent of the patients believed that they were at high risk for developing coronary disease within five years, when in fact three or more risk factors were present in 53 percent of the patients.[25]

Patients with lupus should be advised to stop smoking, to exercise, and to follow measures designed to improve lipid profiles. Hydroxychloroquine should be used in preference to prednisone whenever possible and aspirin should be prescribed for its antiplatelet properties.

Hypertension is an important risk factor in SLE.[40] We favor aggressive therapy, aiming for a diastolic pressure below 85 mmHg, especially in younger patients. The choice of antihypertensive agent depends in part upon coexisting disorders. As examples, we used nifedipine in patients with Raynaud's phenomenon and an angiotensin converting enzyme (ACE) inhibitor in patients with renal disease. Steroids may contribute to hypertension, so the steroid dose should be reduced, if possible.

Symptomatic coronary artery disease should be treated as in patients without lupus.

VENOUS THROMBOSIS

Thrombophlebitis has been reported in approximately 10 percent of patients with SLE.[41] It generally involves the lower extremities, but can also affect the renal veins and inferior vena cava; pulmonary embolism is rare. Risk factors for venous thrombosis include antiphospholipid antibodies and the use of oral contraceptives, particularly in association with smoking cigarettes.

Notes

1. B.F. Mandell, "Cardiovascular involvement in systemic lupus erythematosus." *Semin Arth Rheum* 17 (1987): 126.

2. Roldan, C.A., et al., "Systemic lupus erythematosus valve disease by trans-esophageal echocardiography and the role of antiphospholipid antibodies." *J Am Coll Cardiol* 20 (1992): 1127.

3. Galve, E., et al., "Prevalence, morphologic types, and evolution of cardiac valvular disease in systemic lupus erythematosus." *N Engl J Med* 319 (1988): 817.

4. C.A. Roldan, B.K. Shively, M.H. Crawford, "An echocardiographic study of valvular heart disease associated with systemic lupus erythematosus." *N Engl J Med* 335 (1996): 1424.

5. Cervera, R., et al., "Cardiac disease in systemic lupus erythematosus: Prospective study of 70 patients." *Ann Rheum Dis* 51 (1992):156.

6. G. Sturfelt, J. Eskilsson, O. Nived, "Cardiovascular disease in systemic lupus erythematosus: A study of 75 patients from a defined population." *Medicine* 71 (1992): 216.

7. Hojnik, M., et al., "Heart valve involvement (Libman-Sacks endocarditis) in the antiphospholipid antibody syndrome." *Circulation* 93 (1996): 1579.

8. Khamastha, M.A., et al., "Association of antibodies against phospholipids with heart valve disease in systemic lupus erythematosus." *Lancet* 335 (1990): 1541.

9. Nihoyannopoulos, P., et al., "Cardiac abnormalities in systemic lupus erythematosus. Association with raised anticardiolipin abnormalities." *Circulation* 82 (1990): 369.

10. Barzizza, F., et al., "Mitral valve prolapse in systemic lupus erythematosus." *Clin Exp Rheumatol* 5 (1987): 59.

11. Gabrielli, F., et al. "Cardiac valve involvement in SLE and primary antiphospholipid antibody syndrome: lack of correlation with antiphospholipid antibodies." *Int J Cardiol* 51 (1995): 117.

12. Petri, M., et al., "Plasma homocysteine as a risk factor for atherothrombotic events in systemic lupus erythematosus." *Lancet* 348 (1996): 1120.

13. Zysset, M.K., et al., "Systemic lupus erythematosus: A consideration for antimicrobial prophylaxis." *Oral Surg Oral Med Oral Pathol* 64 (1987): 30.

14. Leung, W.H., et al., "Association between antiphospholipid antibodies and cardiac abnormalities in patients with systemic lupus erythematosus." *Am J Med* 89 (1990): 411.

15. G.G. Hunder, B.J. Mullen, F.C. McDuffie, "Complement in pericardial fluid of lupus erythematosus." *Ann Intern Med* 80 (1974): 453.

16. P.G. Klacsmann, B.H. Bulkley, G.M. Hutchens, "The changed spectrum of purulent pericarditis: An 86 year autopsy experience in 200 patients." *Am J Med* 63 (1977): 666.

17. N.E. Doherty, R.J. Siegel, "Cardiovascular manifestations of systemic lupus erythematosus." *Am Heart J* 110 (1985): 1257.

18. Hochberg, M.C., et al., "Survivorship in systemic lupus erythematosus: Effect of antibody to extractable nuclear antigen." *Arthritis Rheum* 24 (1981): 54.

19. Fairfax, M.J., et al. "Endomyocardial biopsy in patients with systemic lupus erythematosus." *J Rheumatol* 15 (1988): 593.

20. Borenstein, D.G., et al., "The myocarditis of systemic lupus erythematosus." *Ann Intern Med* 89 (1978): 619.

21. Buyon, J.P., et al., "Acquired congenital heart block. Pattern of maternal antibody response to biochemically defined antigens of the SSA/Ro-SSB/La system in neonatal lupus." *J Clin Invest* 84 (1989): 267.

22. Garcia, S., et al., "Cellular mechanism of the conduction abnormalities induced by serum from anti-Ro/SSA-positive patients in rabbit heart." *J Clin Invest* 93 (1994): 718.

23. Guzman, J., et al., "The contribution of resting heart rate and routine blood tests to the clinical assessment of disease activity in systemic lupus erythematosus." *J Rheumatol* 21 (1994): 1845.

24. Rosner, S., et al., "A multicenter study of outcome in systemic lupus erythematosus." *Arthritis Rheum* 25 (1982): 612.

25. Petri, M., et al. "Coronary artery disease risk factors in the Johns Hopkins lupus cohort: Prevalence, recognition by patients, and prevention practices." *Medicine* 71 (1992): 291.

26. J.D. Reveille, A. Bartotucci, G.S. Alarcon, "Prognosis in systemic lupus erythematosus: Negative impact of increasing age at onset, black race, and thrombocytopenia, as well as causes of death." *Arthritis Rheum* 33 (1990): 37.

27. Petri, M., et al., "Risk factors for coronary artery disease in patients with systemic lupus erythematosus." *Am J Med* 93 (1992): 513.

28. A.H. Kutom, H.R. Gibbs, "Myocardial infarction due to intracoronary thrombi without significant coronary disease in systemic lupus erythematosus." *Chest* 100 (1991): 571.

29. L.A. Rubin, M.B. Urowitz, D.D. Gladman, "Mortality in systemic lupus erythematosus—the bimodal pattern revisited." *Q J Med* 55 (1985): 87.

30. H. Johnson, O. Nived, G. Sturfelt, "Outcome in systemic lupus erythematosus: A prospective study of patients from a defined population." *Medicine* 68 (1989):141.

31. Ettinger, W.H., et al., "Dyslipoproteinemia in systemic lupus erythematosus." *Am J Med* 83 (1987): 503.

32. Petri, M., et al., "Effect of prednisone and hydroxychloroquine on coronary risk factors in SLE: A longitudinal data analysis." *Am J Med* 96 (1994): 254.

33. Leong, K.H., et al., "Lipid profiles in patients with systemic lupus erythematosus." *J Rheumatol* 21 (1994): 1264.

34. M.J. Seleznick, J.F. Fries, "Variables associated with decreased survival in SLE." *Semin Arthritis Rheum* 21 (1991): 73.

35. Moroni, G., et al. "Cardiologic abnormalities in patients with long-term lupus nephritis." *Clin Nephrol* 43 (1995): 20.

36. M. Petri, "Thrombosis and systemic lupus erythematosus: The Hopkins Lupus Cohort Perspective." *Scand J Rheumatol* 25 (1996): 191.

37. T. Jouhikainen, S. Pohjola-Sintonen, E. Stephansson, "Lupus anticoagulant and cardiac manifestations in systemic lupus erythematosus." *Lupus* 3 (1994): 167.

38. Greisman, S.G., et al., "Occlusive vasculopathy in systemic lupus erythematosus. Association with anticardiolipin antibody." *Arch Intern Med* 151 (1991): 389.

39. Kabakov, A.E., et al., "The atherogenic effect of lupus sera: Systemic lupus erythematosus-derived immune complexes stimulate the accumulation of cholesterol in cultured smooth muscle cells from human aorta." *Clin Immunol Immunopathol* 63 (1992): 214.

40. Petri, M., et al., "Effect of prednisone and hydroxychloroquine on coronary risk factors in SLE: A longitudinal data analysis." *Am J Med* 95 (1994): 254.

41. D.D. Gladman, M.B. Urowitz, "Venous syndromes and pulmonary embolism in SLE." *Ann Rheum Dis* 39 (1980): 340.

20

Neuropsychiatric Manifestations of Systemic Lupus Erythematosus

by Peter H. Schur, M.D., and Shahram Khoshbin, M.D.

Systemic lupus erythematosus (SLE) may involve the nervous system and present with a number of different neurologic and psychiatric features. The approach to patients with neuropsychiatric symptoms consists of studies that establish the diagnosis of SLE, distinguish between organic and functional etiologies, and exclude symptoms not due to SLE or medications.

Neurologic and psychiatric symptoms occur in 10 to 80 percent of patients, either prior to the diagnosis of the systemic lupus erythematosus (SLE), or during the course of their illnesses. This wide range reflects, in part, the use of different criteria for neuropsychiatric disease. The frequency of neuropsychiatric symptoms appears to be increasing because of both better testing and increased physician awareness.

The neuropsychiatric manifestations of SLE are varied, and may be classified as primary neurologic and psychiatric disease (e.g., related to direct involvement of the nervous system), and secondary disease (e.g., related to complications of the disease and its treatment). The latter is much more common and can be produced by a variety of mechanisms:

- Infections associated with immunosuppressive therapy.

- Metabolic complications of other organ system failure, such as kidney, lung, or heart failure.

- Hypertension.

- Toxic effects of therapy (particularly steroids).

A particular challenge in patients with SLE is to determine whether neurologic symptoms are functional, are due to an organic abnormality, are due to lupus itself (either active or inactive), or are due to other causes.

PATHOPHYSIOLOGY OF NERVOUS SYSTEM INVOLVEMENT

SLE may affect the nervous system at multiple levels, causing different problems. Identification of these diverse pathophysiologic mechanisms has helped to uncover possible mechanisms of immune-mediated neuropsychiatric disorders, and has permitted more accurate and effective therapy.

Nervous system involvement in SLE was initially thought to be due to vasculitis (inflammation of blood vessels). This idea was challenged, however, by investigators who found that true vasculitis in the brain was a rare finding in patients with SLE and neurologic symptoms. Rather, what was found was what has been termed a "vasculopathy," that is a mild inflammation without destruction, which also allows antibodies to cross the blood-brain barrier and enter the brain.

The types of antibodies that have been described and some of their associated clinical features include:

- Antineuronal antibodies targeted to human neuroblastoma cells in 45 percent of patients and in only 5 percent of patients with SLE who did not have nervous system involvement.
- Cognitive dysfunction has been associated with lymphocytotoxic antibodies.
- Antiphospholipid antibodies appear to increase the risk of stroke symptoms.
- Antiribosomal P protein antibodies have been associated with lupus psychosis and depression.
- Antibodies to a 50-kD protein in nineteen of twenty patients with SLE who had CNS involvement; low levels were present in 35 percent of SLE patients without CNS involvement, and this antibody was not detected in normal controls.

A number of factors other than vascular disease and autoantibodies may contribute to CNS lupus. These include cytokines, neuropeptides, and interference with neurotransmission.

The most common neurologic manifestations of SLE are stroke, seizures, headaches, and peripheral neuropathy.

Stroke

Strokes, or cerebrovascular accidents (CVAs), have been reported in up to 15 percent of patients with SLE. Most strokes occurred within the first five years of illness. Stroke syndromes have many potential causes in SLE. Hypertension and accelerated atherosclerosis, both associated with chronic steroid therapy, are common causes of a CVA, as are emboli from the heart that can also block large or small blood vessels.

Patients with antiphospholipid antibodies are at particular risk for developing transient ischemic attacks (TIAs—a disturbance in brain function due to a temporary interruption of the brain's blood supply), stroke with resulting paralysis, sensory loss, visual field defects, difficulty expressing themselves (aphasia), or cognitive defects. An abnormal MRI may be the first clue to the presence of small CVAs and/or antiphospholipid antibodies. Treatment with Coumadin (warfarin) is indicated in most patients with stroke syndromes due to antiphospholipid antibodies or thrombosis once they are stable and if there is no evidence of hemorrhage. The INR is generally maintained between 3 and 4.

Seizures

Seizures occur in approximately 15 to 20 percent of patients with SLE. Generalized convulsions (grand mal) are common, however, partial seizures, both complex (temporal lobe epilepsy), and simple (focal) may be even more common. Seizures may be the first manifestation of lupus or they may develop during the course of the disease.

The causes of seizures are varied and may reflect an acute inflammatory episode or old CNS damage with scarring. Other factors may also contribute, including antiphospholipid antibodies, metabolic disturbances (such as kidney failure), hypertension, infections, tumors, head trauma, stroke, medication withdrawal, vasculopathy, or drug toxicity (e.g., high doses of antimalarials or nitrogen mustard). To establish the cause of seizures, a doctor often performs an MRI of the brain, an EEG, and examination of spinal fluid, as well as blood tests to evaluate lupus activity.

Seizures in patients with CNS lupus are a marker for a poor overall prognosis. However, the seizures can be treated with a variety of medications. Generalized seizures are usually managed with Dilantin (phenytoin) and phenobarbital. Though Dilantin can cause drug-induced lupus, this is not a contraindication for its use in SLE. Partial complex seizures and psychosis related to seizures are best treated with Tegretol (carbamazepine), Klonopin (clonazepam), valproic acid, and the new agent Neurontin (gabapentin). If new onset seizures are thought to reflect an acute inflammatory event, or if a concomitant flare exists, a short course of prednisone (and sometimes immunosuppressives, such as Cytoxan [cyclophosphamide]) may be given in an attempt to prevent the development of a permanent epileptic focus. However, there is no scientific evidence to support this hypothesis.

Headaches

Tension and migraine headaches are frequent complaints in patients with SLE. These headaches may result from numerous causes. Tension or muscle contraction headache is usually triggered by stress, or holding the head and neck (usually during sleep with extra pillows) in a posture that chronically strains the neck and head muscles. Affected patients typically complain of a dull ache, often as a vise encircling the head, as well as a pain in the back of the neck, shoulders, and back of the head.

Migraine headaches have been reported in 10 to 37 percent of patients with SLE, and may be more common than tension headaches. Migraine headaches tend to be severe, persistent, rapid in onset, and mostly one-sided, and are often associated with nausea and vomiting, and light and sound sensations. These headaches frequently occur in the presence of other signs of active lupus, and are often triggered by hormonal changes, oral contraceptives, smoking, stress, alcohol, flashing lights, changes in the weather, or certain foods, such as aged cheese and chocolate. Visual or olfactory symptoms or numbness in a limb may precede the attack. Migraines have been thought to be due to localized blood vessel constriction and dilation, and may be associated with peripheral Raynaud's phenomenon.

Rare but important types and causes of headache include cluster headaches and pseudotumor cerebri with papilledema (a condition that presents symptoms of a tumor in the brain, including intracranial pressure and swelling, without the presence of a tumor. Patients with SLE can also develop headaches due to causes other than lupus, including those precipitated by cold food, hangover, sexual orgasm, nitrites or monosodium glutamate, hunger, sinusitis, dental conditions, and eye diseases. An organic basis for the headaches is suggested by their sudden development in someone previously free of headaches, associated double vision, seizures, or changes in personality.

Patients with SLE tend to be more anxious and depressed than the general population, and may, therefore, be more prone to these headaches.

The treatment of headaches in patients with SLE does not differ from that in patients without this disease unless there are other manifestations of CNS lupus as noted above. Most patients respond to nonsteroid anti-inflammatory drugs (NSAIDs) and/or acetaminophen (Tylenol). Corticosteroids and narcotics are rarely warranted, although they may be beneficial in patients with severe migraines. Tricyclic antidepressants, such as Elavil (amitriptyline), are often helpful for frequently occurring headaches when used at much lower dosages than when they are employed for treatment of depression.

Peripheral Neuropathy

Approximately 10 to 15 percent of patients with SLE develop a peripheral neuropathy (damage to the peripheral nerves) that is probably due to vasculopathy of small arteries supplying the affected nerves. Symptoms are usually asymmetric and mild, may affect more than one nerve, and affect sensory nerves more than motor nerves. A typical presentation may be that of bilateral (but not truly symmetric) tingling and numbness of the fingers or toes, which is often worse at night, that persists for days or weeks; or persistent marked weakness of the toes and feet.

The diagnosis is confirmed by finding abnormalities on nerve conduction studies that differentiate these symptoms from other causes. Neuropathies generally respond to therapy with prednisone.

Uncommon Neurological Syndromes

Movement disorders occur in less than 5 percent of patients. Symptoms may include chorea (repetetive, jerky, uncontrolled movements that may move from one part of the body to another), ataxia (lack of muscular coordination), choreoathetosis (the presence of chorea and athetosis. Athetosis consists of constant involuntary, slow, writhing movements, usually of the hands and feet.), dystonia (involuntary repetetive, slow muscle contractions that may cause the person to "freeze" in the middle of movement), and hemiballismus; there are usually other associated signs of active organic brain involvement. Cranial nerve involvement is usually associated with other manifestations of active SLE. Depending upon the location of the neuropathy, symptoms may include double vision, visual field deficits, trigeminal neuralgia, facial weakness, and vertigo.

Eye involvement in patients with SLE includes a lupus rash of the eyelids, and conjunctivitis (usually infectious). The most characteristic finding is the presence of "cotton wool" exudates (*cytoid bodies*) that are seen with the aid of an ophthalmoscope. Older studies reported that cytoid bodies were found in 10 to 25 percent of patients, usually in association with other manifestations of active lupus; however, these lesions are rare in current practice. Eye movement abnormalities are seen infrequently and are usually transitory. Hearing defects in both low and high frequencies have been noted more frequently in patients with SLE than in the general population.

Transverse myelitis (inflammation of the spinal cord) is rare. Patients present with the sudden onset of lower extremity weakness and/or sensory loss, plus loss of rectal and urinary bladder sphincter control. This syndrome is thought to be due to an arteritis (arterial inflammation), with resultant necrosis (tissue death) of the spinal cord.

Meningitis (manifested by headache, neck rigidity, and cells in the spinal fluid) may develop due to infection, ibuprofen (and other NSAIDs, excluding aspirin), or azathioprine, or without any other apparent cause.

PSYCHIATRIC MANIFESTATIONS

These clinical features are characterized as either diffuse (e.g., coma, depression, and psychosis) or complex (e.g., cognitive disorder with stroke or seizure, and psychiatric presentation with stroke or seizure).

A primary psychiatric disturbance due to CNS lupus is a diagnosis of exclusion; all other possible causes of the observed symptoms, including infection, electrolyte abnormalities, renal failure, drug effects, mass lesions, and arterial emboli must first be eliminated. One clue to the diagnosis is that most acute psychiatric episodes occur during the first two years after the onset of SLE.

The distinction between organic and functional causes of some neuropsychiatric symptoms can occasionally be made by testing for specific autoantibodies. Some investigators believe that antiribosomal P antibodies are associated with lupus psychosis and depression and that cognitive defects (memory, word finding difficulties, attention deficit) are associated with either antineuronal antibodies or antiphospholipid antibodies.

A functional (psychologic) process is assumed in a patient with cognitive defects who has none of these antibodies, a normal neurologic examination, a negative MRI and EEG, and has undergone psychometric testing that "rules out" organic disease.

Psychosis

Psychosis occurs in approximately 5 percent of patients with SLE, usually within the first year of diagnosis. Psychosis is characterized by disordered and bizarre thinking that often includes delusions and hallucinations. Some patients may also present with a fluctuating delirium or "clouding of consciousness," typically occurring at night. Other associated symptoms include a poor attention span, easy distraction, misinterpretation of surroundings, agitation, or combative behavior.

Symptoms may be caused by corticosteroid therapy or, more commonly, by CNS lupus. We have observed that auditory hallucinations are usually caused by steroid therapy, while visual and tactile disturbances are most frequently due to SLE. In the latter circumstance, an association has been noted between lupus psychosis and the presence of antibodies to ribosomal P protein or to neuronal cells. Psychosis due to (active) organic involvement by SLE usually responds to prednisone. If no improvement is seen within two to three weeks, a trial of cytotoxic therapy (e.g., pulse cyclophosphamide—the administration of large amounts of the drug over a short period of time) may be added. While waiting for steroids or immunosuppressive drugs to take effect, psychologic manifestations are best treated with antipsychotic drugs, such as Haldol (haloperidol), as well as with active support by health-care givers and family.

Cognitive Dysfunctions

Cognitive dysfunctions, sometimes referred to as "organic mental syndrome" or "organic brain syndrome," are characterized by any combination of the following symptoms: difficulty with short- or long-term memory, impaired judgment and abstract thinking, aphasia, apraxia (a condition in which one loses the ability to perform tasks that require memory of a sequence of events), agnosia (a condition in which a person cannot associate an object with its usual function), and personality changes. Cognitive defects are relatively common in patients with SLE, with an incidence ranging from 21 percent to 80 percent in studies using tests such as the Stanford-Binet Intelligence test, the Wechsler Adult Intelligence Scale, the Complex Attention Task, and the Pattern Comparison Task.

The following generalizations can be made regarding the clinical and pathophysiologic characteristics of patients with cognitive defects:

- There may be an association with antineuronal or antiphospholipid antibodies.
- Cognitive dysfunction appears to be transient and is not directly correlated with active disease or corticosteroid therapy. However, it is more common in patients with active disease who are receiving corticosteroids.
- Although it may occur independent of psychologic stress, cognitive dysfunction may be caused or exacerbated by a coexistent psychiatric disorder.
- Associated conditions, such as hypertension, multiple small infarcts, and the use of a variety of medications, may produce cognitive dysfunction.
- Focal cerebral dysfunction secondary to neuropsychiatric lupus is probably the cause.

Treatment is based upon the presumed cause of the cognitive abnormalities. If due to medications, such as steroids, consider reducing the dose or stopping therapy. If associated with antiphospholipid antibodies, begin anticoagulant therapy. If associated with antineuronal antibodies, use a short course of prednisone. The use of anticonvulsants and other psychoactive medications is currently under investigation as a treatment. Cognitive retraining may be effective in patients with persistent symptoms.

Dementia

Dementia is characterized by severe cognitive dysfunction, resulting in impaired memory, abstract thinking, and a decreased ability to perform simple manual tasks. The patient may also have difficulty making decisions or controlling impulses.

This syndrome in patients with lupus can reflect multiple small ischemic strokes (due to lack of blood supply) and/or strokes caused by antiphospholipid antibodies.

The exact therapeutic regimen is unclear. Although symptoms occasionally abate without treatment, the following general recommendations can be made. Consideration should be given to discontinuing or lowering the dose of medications that may aggravate symptoms, including nonsteroidal anti-inflammatory drugs (NSAIDs); antimalarial drugs, such as Plaquenil (hydroxychloroquine); antianxiety drugs, such as Valium (diazepam); and corticosteroids. Coexisting depression should be treated by conventional means. Support by family and health professionals, along with reminder prompts, will usually help patients deal with this problem.

SECONDARY PSYCHIATRIC MANIFESTATIONS

Although depression, anxiety, and manic behavior may occasionally reflect organic involvement, these symptoms are more typically functional. The distinction between organic and functional disease is based upon a psychiatric interview, psychological testing, and other studies that may include CT scan, magnetic resonance imaging (MRI), single photon emission compound tomography (SPECT) scans, evoked potentials, electroencephalograms (EEG), and cerebrospinal fluid analysis.

The specific psychologic symptoms that occur may include phobias, depression, anxiety, mania, headaches, mood swings, agoraphobia with and without panic, social phobia, alcohol abuse, or cognitive problems, such as poor concentration, impaired memory, and difficulty with word finding or spatial orientation. The individual pattern that develops usually reflects the patient's coping mechanisms used to deal with the stress of chronic illness, rather than a specific disease process.

Interactions between the patient and physician can occasionally adversely affect symptom resolution. Patients often relate a long history of frustration in obtaining the proper diagnosis, and physicians find that evaluating patients who have symptoms and signs suggesting a cognitive impairment is difficult.

Depression

The most common psychologic symptom in patients with SLE is depression. Depressive symptoms usually begin acutely. They reflect the patient's reaction to chronic illness and the significant lifestyle limitations that must be endured, including difficulties with pregnancy, fatigue, limited sun exposure, and chronic medication use. There may also be an organic basis in some cases. Some depressed patients, for example, have elevated levels of certain autoantibodies or are more prone to have associated illnesses. An association has been reported between severe depression and antiribosomal P antibodies, but not with other antibodies.

Most patients recover within one year with the help of family, friends, physicians, and/or other professionals. Other patients may incorporate the depression into their personality, thereby developing many concurrent (psycho)somatic complaints, such as insomnia, anorexia, constipation, myalgia, arthralgia, and fatigue. Patients may also develop "psychotic" features, with increasing despair, loss of hope, and even suicidal tendencies; prompt psychiatric intervention is essential in this circumstance.

Anxiety

Following the initial diagnosis of SLE, or after an acute exacerbation, some patients display symptoms of anxiety, either instead of or in addition to depression. The patient may become anxious about a variety of possible consequences of their illness, including disfigurement, disability, dependency, loss of a job, social isolation, or death.

Anxiety may be manifested by heart palpitations; diarrhea; sweating; hyperventilation; dizzy spells; difficulty with speech, memory, or words; fear of "going crazy"; or headaches. This state may deteriorate into obsessive-compulsive behavior, phobias, hypochondriasis, sleep disturbances, and a reduction in social contacts and interaction.

Other Psychiatric Manifestations

Some patients develop manic behavior or an organic personality disorder. The former is characterized by a marked increase in energy and activity, irritability, and sleeplessness. This behavior is usually due to high doses of steroids. A sudden marked change in personality may also occur due to any of the causes discussed above, with symptoms including apathy, indifference, emotional liability, sexual indiscretions, verbosity, religiosity, and/or aggressiveness. Psychiatric abnormalities may be secondary to a primary psychiatric disorder (e.g., bipolar disorder) or to psychological stress associated with a chronic and potentially lethal disease.

TESTING FOR CNS INVOLVEMENT IN LUPUS

Although it would be desirable to have diagnostic tests that establish a specific diagnosis of neuropsychiatric lupus, such tests do not exist. This problem is further compounded by the multiple ways that neuropsychological lupus can express itself. However, there are tests that may help a doctor determine whether or not certain symptoms are due to the effects of lupus on the central nervous system.

Blood Tests

Blood tests are typically used to help establish the diagnosis of SLE. Antinuclear antibodies (ANAs) are positive in virtually all patients with this disorder. However, the presence of ANA is not a very specific finding, and many non-SLE patients have symptoms such as headache or fatigue with only a weakly positive ANA.

Serum levels of anti-DNA and anti-Sm antibodies and low levels of complement are useful in this setting to corroborate the diagnosis of SLE.

In the patient with established SLE, an association between neuropsychiatric symptoms and detection of specific antibodies has been demonstrated by some in three circumstances:

• Antiribosomal P antibodies have been associated with psychosis and severe depression.

- Antiphospholipid antibodies have been associated with cerebrovascular accidents, multi-infarct dementia, seizures, deep-vein and cortical sinus thromboses, chorea, and transverse myelitis.

- Antineuronal antibodies are found in some, but not all patients with cognitive dysfunction.

Psychological Testing

Psychometric testing is extremely useful in helping to differentiate functional from organic disease. These tests should be supplemented with a psychiatric interview.

Cerebrospinal Fluid Analysis

Routine evaluation of the cerebrospinal fluid (CSF) is usually normal in patients with CNS lupus, except in cases of aseptic meningitis and transverse myelitis. Some reports, however, have noted immunologic abnormalities including elevated levels of anti-DNA antibodies, immunoglobulin G (IgG—a class of antibodies), oligoclonal banding, immune complexes, and interleukin-6, which may roughly correlate with neuropsychiatric disease.

Electroencephalography

Approximately 80 percent of patients with active CNS lupus will have an abnormal routine EEG. Diffuse slow wave activity is the pattern most typically associated with mental state abnormalities, while focal changes are seen in patients with seizure disorders or focal neurological problems. The specificity of the EEG, however, is not as high as its sensitivity, since abnormal electroencephalograms have also been noted in patients without apparent CNS lupus for some specific cognitive disabilities. Evoked potentials and evoked potential mapping may be even more sensitive in detecting abnormalities.

Imaging Studies

A number of imaging methods are available for use in the diagnosis of neuropsychiatric SLE. Computed tomography (CT scanning) and particularly magnetic resonance imaging (MRI) are the most useful. CT scans are useful for detecting structural and focal abnormalities (such as infarcts, hemorrhage, tumors). Brain atrophy has been noted in some patients; this finding has been thought by some (but disputed by others) to reflect the effects of steroid therapy or age. We have seen brain atrophy out of proportion to a patient's age, and prior to steroid therapy.

MRI is more sensitive than CT, and may reveal abnormalities that reflect focal neuropsychiatric lupus. However, MRI may also reveal white matter lesions or periventricular hyperintensities in patients with SLE who do not have neuropsychiatric symptoms. These white matter abnormalities may be difficult to interpret since they are present in 20 percent of the population younger than age 50, and in 90 percent of people older than age 70. The value of MRI in CNS lupus is still under investigation.

Single photon emission computed tomography (SPECT) scanning has been advocated by some to be more sensitive than MRI for detecting brain abnormalities in patients with SLE. However, this test is also frequently abnormal in patients without CNS lupus.

Angiography has been used historically to demonstrate vasculitis. However, magnetic resonance angiography is rapidly becoming as sensitive in demonstrating these lesions.

31P NMR spectroscopy has been used to monitor changes in ATP and phosphocreatine during acute episodes of CNS lupus, and proton NMR has been used to study anatomic changes in the brains of SLE patients with brain atrophy. Experience is limited with these techniques.

Positron emission tomography (PET), using radio-labeled oxygen to assess brain cell metabolism and radio-labeled CO_2 to evaluate cerebral vascular blood flow, has demonstrated abnormalities of cell metabolism and regional blood flow in patients with SLE. This test is expensive, however, and not readily available.

Radionuclide brain scanning is generally not useful.

The preceding discussion has primarily emphasized the use of specific therapy for different forms of neurologic manifestations of SLE. This may or may not include the use of corticosteroids. The role of cyclophosphamide and/or plasmapheresis in the management of CNS lupus is not well defined. We recommend cyclophosphamide when a patient with inflammatory organic brain symptoms has failed to respond to a one to two week course of high-dose oral corticosteroids.

21

The Antiphospholipid (Hughes') Syndrome— "Thick Blood"

by Graham R.V. Hughes, M.D., F.R.C.P.

A CASE HISTORY

A 41-year-old woman complained of recurring headaches and memory loss. She had frequently driven past the entrance to her own street on her way home. In the past, she had suffered frequent migraines, had had a leg vein thrombosis when she was in her twenties, and had had four failed pregnancies, all ending in spontaneous abortion.

Her blood tests were unremarkable, apart from showing a positive anticardiolipin test. Brain scan (MRI) showed a number of small white spots suggestive of impaired blood flow. She was treated with Coumadin (warfarin—a blood thinning agent. The headaches ceased, and over the following months there was a striking improvement in her memory.

In 1982 I presented clinical details of a new syndrome at the British Society of Rheumatology (Heberden Round) and the American College of Rheumatology. Between 1983 and 1985, my research group and I went on to publish a series of papers describing the tendency of those afflicted with this syndrome toward artery and vein thrombosis, brain disease, recurrent miscarriages, low platelets, pulmonary hypertension, epilepsy, and skin rashes (livedo).

We showed that this new syndrome, now frequently known as "sticky blood," was very strikingly associated with a blood antibody called *anticardiolipin* or *antiphospholipid* antibody.

We set up standard tests for the antibody, and in 1985 held the first "world" conference and workshop on the syndrome—a distinctly local affair despite its grand title. Our work was taken up internationally by groups in Holland, Mexico, the United States, Italy, France, and Australia.

Our early studies were in lupus but it very quickly became clear that many of the patients did not have classical lupus. We, therefore, introduced the name anticardiolipin syndrome, a name we changed in 1985 to the "primary antiphospholipid syndrome." At the 5th international meeting in Leuven in 1995, a number of colleagues renamed the disease Hughes' Syndrome.

CLINICAL FEATURES

The main feature is "sticky blood"—a tendency for the blood to clot too easily. This can affect veins or arteries in any part of the body, causing an almost limitless list of features. The more common features are deep vein thrombosis (DVTs— sometimes on starting the oral contraceptive pill), headaches and migraine, memory loss, shortness of breath (lung clots and heart valve disease), or, in pregnancy, thrombosis of the placenta and recurrent fetal loss.

While almost any limb or organ can be affected by thrombosis, the brain seems to be particularly frequently involved. The degree of involvement can be from relatively "minor" headaches, flashing lights, and memory disturbances, to more serious manifestations, such as seizures, transient strokes, and major strokes.

Many women with the syndrome give a history of recurrent spontaneous abortion—often as late as halfway through the pregnancy. In many individuals, this is the only outward sign of the presence of antiphospholipid antibodies.

We are not sure why this clotting occurs. Collaborative international research is underway to look at ways in which the antibodies cause trouble. Possible mechanisms include effects on clotting proteins, on blood platelets (in some patients the actual number or circulating platelets falls), and on the lining of the blood vessels themselves. The more fundamental question—Why are the antibodies produced in the first place?—is also unanswered.

TREATMENT

Now that many of these patients' problems have been recognized as being caused by "sticky blood," anticoagulants (either "junior" aspirin, Coumadin, or heparin) are the logical choice. For many, many patients, the successes have been enormous. For example, in our lupus pregnancy clinic at St. Thomas' Hospital, the pregnancy success rate for patients with the syndrome has changed from less than 20 percent ten years ago to nearly 80 percent now.

For the physician, the recognition and management of these patients has proved one of the most satisfying experiences in the whole of medicine.

22

S.L.E. *and Genetics*

by Robert B. Zurier, M.D.

Systemic lupus erythematosus (SLE) is an autoimmune disease in which autoantibodies can damage multiple organ systems and cause a variety of clinical manifestations. A hallmark of the disease is the accumulation of immunoglobulin G (IgG) antibodies, caused by their increased production and reduced clearance from the body. These IgG, or so-called antinuclear, antibodies attack the nuclei of certain cells.

A considerable body of evidence indicates that SLE has a strong genetic basis. For example, studies of families suggest that a patient's sibling has a twentyfold increased risk of developing SLE compared with the general population, and, despite this increase, the sibling's absolute risk is still only one in twenty. In addition, the concordance rate for SLE in identical twins has been estimated to be about 25 percent compared with about 2 percent in fraternal twins.

As new knowledge of the genetics of the immune response are discovered, associations of SLE with genetic markers—such as increased frequencies of certain human leukocyte antigens and hereditary deficiencies of complement components—are becoming apparent. At the same time, the clinical heterogeneity of lupus is being recognized, and a number of disease subsets, associated mainly with different autoantibody profiles, are now being defined. Recent advances in molecular biology now make it possible to examine these genetic associations at a more basic level. New methods allow for the identification of the chromosomal location of genes linked with a disease or a particular manifestation of the disease.

Lupus is a generally heterogeneous disease comprising several overlapping autoimmune responses, and many different genes contribute to susceptibility to SLE. In about 5 percent of patients, a single gene may be responsible for the disease manifestations. For the other 95 percent of patients with SLE, multiple genes are required. Some authorities estimate that a minimum of three or four and possibly as many as six susceptibility genes are required. Studies of inbred mouse strains that develop SLE-like disease suggest that the number of susceptibility genes required may be greater than ten. In addition, one gene may influence each disease feature, such as nephritis, anti-double stranded DNA antibodies, and hyperactivity of B and T lymphocytes. Thus, no one particular gene is necessary or sufficient for disease expression.

How do genes predispose to SLE? When this question is answered fully, we will understand the syndromes that collectively fulfill the criteria for SLE. The identification of multiple predisposing genes, which is bound to occur in the next decade, is sure to provide greater insight into an understanding of the abnormal immune responses that lead to tissue injury and organ damage in patients with SLE.

23

How Systemic Lupus Erythematosus Affects the Blood

by Elizabeth Petri Henske, M.D.

There are three types of cells found in the blood: red blood cells, which carry oxygen; white blood cells, which fight infection; and platelets, which are an important component of blood clots. Systemic lupus erythematosus (SLE) can cause low counts in all three types of blood cells. Fortunately, the low counts are usually not severe and treatment is available.

HOW DOES SLE AFFECT RED BLOOD CELLS?

Anemia, a condition in which there are too few red blood cells, is common in those with SLE. Symptoms of anemia can include fatigue and shortness of breath, but often the anemia of SLE is not severe enough to cause any specific symptoms.

Anemia of chronic disease (ACD) is the most common type of anemia in individuals with SLE. In ACD, the bone marrow does not make enough red blood cells. The reason for this is not yet understood. ACD also occurs in individuals with cancer and chronic infections. Unfortunately, there is no specific treatment for ACD, but it usually improves when the underlying disease (such as SLE) improves.

Anemia in individuals with SLE can also be caused by autoimmune hemolytic anemia (AIHA). In AIHA, the bone marrow makes adequate numbers of red cells, but they are being destroyed because of a mistaken response from the patient's own immune system to red blood cells. AIHA is often treated with prednisone.

Iron deficiency is an important cause of anemia in individuals with SLE. It can be caused by blood loss through the gastrointestinal tract or through heavy menstrual blood flow. Iron-deficiency anemia is treated with iron tablets.

Sometimes anemia in SLE is caused by a combination of these conditions. Measuring the blood levels of iron and iron-binding proteins, testing the blood for red cell antibodies, and examining the size and shape of the red cells under a microscope are three important studies that identify these types of anemia so they can be treated.

HOW DOES SLE AFFECT PLATELETS?

Thrombocytopenia, or a low platelet count, is common in SLE, but fortunately it does not usually cause symptoms. If the platelet count is very low, nose bleeds, heavy menstrual blood flow, and bruising of the skin can occur.

Thrombocytopenia in SLE is usually caused by immune thrombocytopenic purpura (ITP). In this condition, antibodies in the blood cause the platelets to be destroyed. This is similar to what occurs in AIHA, in which the antibodies bind to red cells. ITP, like AIHA, is often treated with prednisone.

HOW DOES SLE AFFECT WHITE BLOOD CELLS?

Leukopenia, or a low white cell count, can occur in individuals with SLE, but fortunately it is usually not severe enough to interfere with the body's ability to fight infection. Leukopenia, like ITP and AIHA, is sometimes caused by antibodies.

SLE can cause all three types of cells in the blood, the red cells, the white cells, and the platelets, to decrease to low levels. These conditions, which can be diagnosed with blood tests, are often not severe enough to cause symptoms, and if they do cause symptoms are usually treatable.

24

Skin Rashes in Lupus Erythematosus

by Dr. Carmen G. Espinoza

Over the past ten years, I have interviewed Dr. Luis Espinoza, a Professor of Medicine and Chief of Rheumatology in the Department of Medicine at Louisiana State University Medical School, and he has written several articles for Lupus News. On one of my visits to New Orleans, after I met with Luis Espinoza, he introduced me to his wife, Dr. Carmen Espinoza, who is also a physician and a Professor of Pathology at the same medical school as her husband.

Meeting with Dr. Carmen Espinoza was a delightful and enriching experience. She is a pleasant, attractive woman endowed with a gift of laughter and the warmth of a mother. She speaks proudly of her two children—both in medical schools, following in the footsteps of their parents. Dr. Carmen Espinoza spoke of her interest in the often neglected clinical manifestations of lupus with skin involvement. She was concerned because some of the overlapping features of rashes confuse many patients, and even some physicians. "Patients need to know about the multitude of lupus-related rashes and to be alerted to the seriousness of a rash or lesion. These rashes should not be confused with sun poisoning, drug reactions, or other causes," she said.

Talking with her, I recalled when, in the early 1950s, my facial rash was confused with a severe sunburn and sun poisoning. This was a long time ago, but it is apparent that misdiagnoses still occur, despite today's knowledge and awareness of lupus.

I showed Dr. Espinoza a mark on my right calf, the remainder of a blister I had prior to coming to New Orleans. The blister had been the size of an egg and full of clear fluid—a scary and unpleasant sight. My doctor had told me not to puncture the blister, which he believed had been caused by a nasty spider bite. Dr. Carmen Espinoza thought otherwise. She showed me a picture of a blister identical to mine, a manifestation of bullous lupus erythematosus, which is characterized by blisters similar to mine. "Such blisters can occur after unprotected exposure to the sun," she said, and, indeed, I remembered that prior to the appearance of the blister, I had tended to my flower pots on the porch, barefoot under a blazing hot sun.

Dr. Carmen Espinoza's comments raised new questions in my mind. I have been in a complete remission for over twenty years. And I suddenly asked myself whether I could still have a predisposition to lupus. If so, did I have to use precautions, as *if I still had active disease? And I further asked myself, what role does preventative medicine play in people with a history of an abnormal immune system? I am aware that I'm still susceptible to infections, and I still have some pains and aches, and I still feel tired—sometimes I feel dead tired. I am still allergic to some medications and foods; and the sun, obviously, is still my enemy. Even though my lupus tests have been negative for all those years, could I still have a mild form of lupus? Those were questions for me to think about, and at some point in time, discuss with my physician.*

Before I parted with the Doctors Espinoza, Dr. Carmen Espinoza promised to send me an article on skin rashes in lupus erythematosus. Here is what she wrote:

Lupus erythematosus is a multisystemic, chronic, inflammatory disorder of unknown cause, that affects preferentially women in their childbearing age. The skin is one of the most common systems affected in patients with systemic lupus erythematosus, with a prevalence of 59 percent; and often times is the presenting manifestation. Because of the low mortality associated with skin involvement, this clinical manifestation is often neglected and/or confused with a multitude of non-specific rashes. Lupus erythematosus has a broad spectrum of skin manifestations, some of them with overlapping features. One of the most important characteristics of lupus rash is its propensity for photosensitivity; in other words, sun exposure aggravates a preexisting lupus rash or triggers it anew. In general, any type of skin rash can be seen in lupus erythematosus patients. The skin lesions specific for lupus erythematosus are classified based on morphological features and sympto-matology. The aim of this article is to describe the appearance of some of the specific cutaneous lesions, and some other lesions that are not specific but when present may be associated with systemic lupus erythematosus.

SPECIFIC SKIN RASH IN LUPUS ERYTHEMATOSUS

The cutaneous findings described as specific may be seen in different clinical settings, but, in general, acute cutaneous lupus and bullous lupus erythematosus usually are associated with systemic lupus erythematosus; subacute cutaneous lupus may be associated with musculoskeletal system involvement but only rarely involve other organs; and chronic cutaneous lupus erythematosus may be limited to skin, but is one of the criteria for SLE. Lupus panniculitis may be associated with discoid lupus or SLE.

Acute Cutaneous Lupus Erythematosus

Acute cutaneous lupus erythematosus usually presents as an erythematous rash in a butterfly distribution on the face. This blush is slightly swollen and is located on both cheeks and across the bridge of the nose. The lesion usually appears after sun exposure but persists a few days to weeks before healing without scarring. It may be accompanied by erythematous lesions in other areas of the body.

Usually more than 90 percent of the cases have positive ANA, and immunoglobulin deposits along the dermoepidermal junction can be detected by immunofluorescence studies of involved skin, and in 75 percent of uninvolved skin.

Subacute Cutaneous Lupus Erythematosus Lesions

Subacute cutaneous lupus erythematosus lesions may be localized or generalized. The maculopapular rash usually occurs after sun exposure. The lesions are usually itchy. It may involve any place on the body, and, because the erythematous lesions may involve palms and soles, they resemble a drug reaction. The great majority of these lesions heal without scarring; however, persistent lesions that become crusty may heal with only slight atrophy of the skin. This type of rash is associated with a high prevalence (70 percent) of Ro (SS-A) antibodies; however, only 50 percent of cases have positive immunoglobulin deposition in lesional skin when immunofluoresced.

Chronic Cutaneous Lupus Erythematosus

Chronic cutaneous lupus erythematosus, referred to as discoid lupus erythematosus, usually involves the face, scalp, and ears, but it may occur anywhere. The rash may itch. The lesions at the beginning are red, slightly elevated papules or plaques, that in time become raised, bright red, and swollen. Later on, the center becomes depressed and the color fades and becomes atrophic, while the swollen red periphery slowly enlarges and becomes irregular with some dilation of capillaries. In older lesions, follicular plugging, characterized by small round areas of hyperkeratosis (an overgrowth of dead skin cells), are noted. Later on, the lesions heal with a scar, leaving a white area with or without hyperpigmentation. In lesion of the scalp where the lesions are red and scaly, the hair usually grows back, but if the lesion heals with scarring, the loss of hair in that area is permanent.

The name of the different variants reflects the predominant component of the lesion; the tumidus, for example, refers to raised lesions that are peculiarly soft to the touch, as the feeling to the touch obtained compressing a cotton ball.

Only 5 to 10 percent of cases of those with this type of rash have a positive ANA, and immunoglobulin deposits at the dermoepidermal junction are present in 80 percent of involved skin by immunofluorescence studies, but usually immunofluorescence studies are negative in lesions less than 3 months old.

Lupus Panniculitis

Lupus panniculitis, also known as lupus profundus, appears as deep nodules. The lesions are situated below the skin in the subcutaneous tissue and heals with a deep atrophy of the involved area.

Bullous Lupus Erythematosus

Bullous lupus erythematosus is characterized by the presence of blisters, which contain a clear serous fluid, and may range from 3 to 4 millimeters in diameter. The rash usually appears in sun exposed areas, and only rarely is associated with burning sensation, mild itching, or redness. Some papules may accompany the blisters. The lesion may resolve spontaneously usually without scar after a week, but they reappear episodically.

Neonatal Lupus

Neonatal lupus is seen in newborn babies, and the rash is similar to the annular-polycyclic rash seen in subacute lupus erythematosus, with widespread distribution. Occasionally, a baby presents with lesions similar to those of discoid lupus erythematosus. Mothers with Ro (SS-A) positivity with or without lupus may have babies with neonatal lupus. These mothers also share increased frequency of HLA-B8, HLA-DR3, HLA-DQ23, and HLA-DRw52 phenotypes.

MORPHOLOGICAL FEATURES OF NONSPECIFIC SKIN LESIONS

There are several different types of skin lesions that are not specific to lupus. These are described below.

Urticarial Vasculitis

Urticarial vasculitis presents as hives (circumscribed redness and swelling). It usually itches, which lasts more than twenty-four to seventy-two hours. Severe cases resemble leukocytoclastic vasculitis.

Leukocytoclastic Vasculitis

Leukocytoclastic vasculitis presents as palpable purpura characterized by red papules, usually symmetric with predilection for lower extremities. Some of the lesions may evolve into hemorrhagic blisters and infarcts.

Thrombosis Without Vasculitis

Thrombosis without vasculitis may resemble leukocytoclastic vasculitis, and may be seen in patients with antiphospholipid antibodies.

Telogen Effluvium

Telogen effluvium refers to the diffuse loss of hair for one or two months, usually following a marked disturbance of general physiology. Many patients report this type of hair loss after having a baby. Complete regrowth is the rule, provided the original insult is not prolonged or repeated.

DIFFERENTIAL DIAGNOSIS

It is important to remember that patients with lupus erythematosus may have other skin processes, and numerous cutaneous rashes due to other causes may resemble the rash of lupus erythematosus. The most common rashes that may have a butterfly distribution in the face and are not lupus erythematosus, include chronic polymorphous light eruption, seborrheic dermatitis, early psoriasis of the sun-sensitive area, and acne rosacea. Lesions in other areas that are confused with lupus erythematosus includes lichen planus, tinea, and sarcoidosis. Since all of these have histopathological features different from the ones in lupus, a biopsy will help to establish the correct diagnosis. Sometimes drug reactions must have histological features identical to that of lupus erythematosus. See the end of this article for a reference for the latest update in lupus erythematosus.

THERAPY

Fortunately, most rashes associated with the systemic form of lupus erythematosus respond to topical steroid therapy. Salicilates and other nonsteroid anti-inflammatory agents control the mild pain that may accompany the skin rash.

Most rashes respond to antimalarials. Occasionally, systemic steroid therapy—mild to moderate doses—will be required to control the rash. The rash usually heals without leaving scars.

The subacute and chronic forms of cutaneous lupus are more difficult to manage. In these situations, a judicious use of topical corticosteroid creams, and the use of systemic antimalarial agents have proven to be of great benefit. Intralesional steroid injection of chronic discoid lupus lesions may be necessary at times. It is important to establish a good rapport with affected patients, and avoid unnecessary long-term use of oral and/or topical steroids. Sunscreens as a preventive measure and cosmetics are also useful to patients. If the suspected rash fails to respond to adequate therapeutic management, a skin biopsy may prove to be very useful. Acne rosacea, for example, often shows to be extremely difficult to distinguish from lupus; it may adopt an identical appearance—butterfly distribution, but fails to respond to anti-inflammatory therapy and tends to affect older women.

25

Ultraviolet Light and the Immune System

by Henrietta Aladjem
in Conversation With Luis R. Espinoza, M.D.

According to Dr. Espinoza, "One of the most well-known environmental factors affecting patients with systemic lupus erythematosus (SLE) is sunlight or, specifically, ultraviolet light." He explained that 25 to 40 percent of lupus patients report having been overexposed to sun before the onset of disease. Furthermore, a rash after sun exposure, or photosensitivity, may elicit any type of skin rash, including the classic butterfly rash. In addition, photosensitivity may also exacerbate some of the systemic manifestations of lupus, including those of the kidney.

"Sunlight affects almost every aspect of human life and is vital for our survival," he said. "Solar radiation provides the energy necessary for our food chains and climate, yet it has profound effects on the immune system that may eventually lead to dysfunction and disease." He explained that ultraviolet radiation (UVR) belongs to a specific region (200 to 400 nm) of the electromagnetic spectrum. This area has been further subdivided into three subregions termed UVC (200 to 280 nm), UVB (290 to 320 nm), and UVA (320 to 400 nm). At the surface of the earth, UVA radiation is found in large quantities. UVA can induce increased melanin production but is weak at inducing redness of the skin. UVB radiation penetrates the atmosphere in large amounts and induces redness, or erythema, of the skin. UVC radiation also induces skin redness, but its penetration to the surface of the earth is blocked by a layer of ozone. The ozone layer acts as a shield, protecting the earth's surface against detrimental radiation. All UVC and some UVB radiation is normally blocked by the ozone layer, while UVA radiation is not affected. However, the ozone layer's degradation, which has been documented, has allowed increased UVB radiation to reach the earth's surface in the past several years, and may eventually lead to deleterious effects for human life.

Once UV radiation comes into contact with skin, it is absorbed into important biomolecules, such as DNA. Most of its deleterious effects occur as a result of its action on DNA. He spoke about the clinical side effects of ultraviolet radiation, including the following possibilities:

- Photosensitivity or rashes in lupus and other connective tissue disorders.
- Exacerbation of lupus disease activity.
- Triggering the onset of lupus.

- Skin aging.
- Skin cancer, especially basal cell and squamous cell cancers, and malignant melanoma.
- Interaction with medications in the skin, e.g., NSAIDs and Plaquenil (hydroxychloroquine).

He also explained the mechanisms of action of UVR-induced lupus rash and of disease exacerbation, and said that lupus patients with positive Ro/SSA autoantibodies are more prone to the development of photosensitivity. It has been recently established that exposure to UV radiation results in the expression of Ro/SSA antigen on the surfaces of skin cells. Once Ro/SSA antigen is expressed, it binds circulating Ro/SSA antibody, and the resulting bound antibody triggers cutaneous lesions by antibody-directed cell cytotoxicity. Evidence also suggests that UV radiation triggers programmed cell death, leading to exposure of cell nuclear material, which also binds to circulating autoantibodies, including Ro/SSA.

"UV radiation can also induce exacerbation of the symptoms of lupus in a significant proportion of patients (up to 40 percent)," he said, and went on to explain that the exact mechanism is unclear, but may also involve profound perturbation of the immune system and UV-induced expression of nuclear antigens on the surface of skin cells. Experimental work suggests that UV radiation may exacerbate lupus activity through activation of helper T-lymphocytes. UVB irradiation has been shown to activate helper T-lymphocytes, thereby stimulating B-cell activity. B-cell hyperactivity is one of the most prominent immunological abnormalities seen in lupus patients, and an unrestrained helper T-lymphocyte activity may explain this finding. In contrast, UVA irradiation does not appear to have this harmful side effect. On the contrary, as it has been recently shown, UVA irradiation may decrease clinical disease activity and autoantibodies in some patients with systemic lupus erythematosus.

He also touched upon UV radiation and skin cancer. He said that evidence accumulated over the past several years has conclusively shown that UV radiation induces perturbation of the immune system leading to the development of malignant disease (cancer) of the skin. Exposure to UV-B radiation *in vivo* depresses the functions of Langerhans cells normally residing in the skin, suppresses the induction of contact and delayed hypersensitivity, increases circulating cytokine (interleukin-1) activity, and alters the proportion of lymphocyte subsets in the circulation, leading to suppression of the normal immune response and facilitation of the growth of skin cancer.

He pointed out that epidemiologic data supports the above described mechanisms. First of all, skin cancer in humans is correlated with long-term cumulative exposure to sunlight. Furthermore, it also has been shown that immunosuppressed persons have a marked increase in the rate of skin cancer.

"In conclusion," he said, "UV radiation is fundamental for human life. However, overexposure to it leads to deleterious or harmful side effects ranging from photosensitivity in lupus patients to the development of skin cancer."

26

Lupus and Fatigue

by Robert S. Schwartz, M.D.

At a training session for claim examiners and physicians in the Social Security Disability Services Program in Boston, a few lupus patients described their experiences with fatigue, and Dr. Robert S. Schwartz spoke about the excruciating lupus fatigue and his interest in this particular symptom. He later wrote a story entitled "Fatigue and the Vexed Lupus Patient," which appeared in A Decade of Lupus *and* Lupus News. *Here is what Dr. Schwartz wrote:*

Four years ago, when February's blasts were rattling the bedroom windows, I, too, was shaking. But my chills were not of the wintry kind; the fever and drenching sweats convinced me of that. Too sick that night to think about diagnostic possibilities, I waited for the clarifying effect of morning. But even then, the reason for my malaise was not apparent. So it was off to the doctor! He didn't see its cause either. After conducting several tests and taking blood samples, he returned me to the rattling windows for another night of the chills. By the next morning, the problem was obvious. As I gazed at the yellow-stained eyes in the mirror, the phone rang.

"Guess what?" the doctor said.

"I know," I responded.

"Hepatitis," he said.

"Yeah."

"Bad hepatitis," he told me.

"I know." I crawled back for two more weeks.

When February's ice relented, so did the itching of my saffron skin. By March I moved out of the bed to the couch to "convalesce." I developed an inexplicable and insatiable desire for eggs—poached eggs. Breakfast: poached eggs; lunch: poached eggs; supper: poached eggs. Then it began. A peculiar weariness set in, usually after the fourth egg. Lethargy to the point of exhaustion. Loss of interest. Fatigue. It certainly couldn't have been the physical act of ingesting a few eggs. I couldn't understand why I was feeling so rundown when I should have been feeling better. All of my tests were normal.

I decided to return to work. The mail was piling up. Telephone messages made pink dunes on my desk. The first day was finished for me after only two hours.

Wilted, I took a taxi home to collapse on the couch, crushed by fatigue. I slept twelve hours a day. By April I could work three, then four, then six hours a day. May brought its tulips, and with them came new energy and that ambition. I was back. The fatigue was over.

It was hard to forget. I thought about my patients and their fatigue. I realized that at last I understood—really understood—what they were trying to tell me about how they felt, about how their lives were changed by whatever it was that ended their day at 3:00 in the afternoon. And I began to examine the problem so that I could comprehend better. I broke fatigue down into three categories—early morning lassitude, late morning-early afternoon exhaustion, and twilight apathy. Each type of fatigue seemed to carry with it a different motif.

Twilight Apathy

Twilight apathy, or evening fatigue, it seemed to me, was perfectly normal. After all, I myself had had it for years. It consists of reclining on the sofa with a newspaper, usually around 6:00 or 7:00 in the evening, and within about five minutes, falling into a most pleasant state of relaxation. The newspaper slips to the floor. After fifteen or twenty minutes, I awaken to hear, "Dinner is ready!" Refreshed, I eat. The only side effect of an excess of this agreeable habit is insomnia: If I oversleep before dinner, a state of alertness later that night is to be expected.

Early Morning Lassitude

By contrast, early morning lassitude is not normal—unless one has been up all night. But given six to eight hours of restful nighttime sleep, the alarm bell should bring with it a sense of readiness for the day, at least by the first cup of coffee. Persistent morning fatigue lasting for hours, and sometimes for the entire day, is abnormal. I am not including in this category those conditions with other symptoms that could account for the weariness, such as the morning stiffness of rheumatoid arthritis, or obvious organic disorders that produce weakness of muscles. Nor do I count here the occasional feeling of fatigue as a normal response to overwork. What I am discussing is persistent, day in-day out lassitude that is uncorrected by appropriate rest, is relentless despite a normal pattern of sleep, is unrelated to one's labor, and is apparent in the morning and continuing stubbornly throughout most of the day. A patient with this symptom is most likely depressed.

All too often, unfortunately, the suggestion of depression as a cause of this form of fatigue is rejected by the patient, who prefers a real diagnosis—as if "depression" was only a metaphor reinforcing the sense of unworthiness that brought on the symptom in the first place. But depression is a legitimate illness and a treatable one. Anyone can become depressed, even a patient with lupus, a development that demands the most careful evaluation of fatigue in that disease. Here is an example of a recent problem I encountered:

A 30-year-old woman consulted a dermatologist because of a red, scaly rash on her cheeks. The diagnosis of lupus erythematosus of the skin was established by clinical examination and biopsy of the rash. She also complained of marked fatigue, so she was referred for a complete medical evaluation. Careful questioning revealed fatigue of the type I have been discussing. The symptom was severe enough to cause her to leave her job in a law office. Apart from the facial rash, the examination was normal. All laboratory tests were normal, including tests for systemic lupus erythematosus and low thyroid function.

More medical and social history was obtained. The patient is a virtual recluse. She has neither friends nor social life. She rarely leaves the house. While in college, a psychological evaluation was done for reasons she was reluctant to disclose. The possibility of depression was raised but firmly rejected. Offers to arrange a second psychological interview were turned down. The physician's appeal to a close relative was ineffective.

The patient continued her secluded life, worn down by her depression, unwilling to accept help. Her fatigue was unrelated to lupus, however: she has the localized discoid form of the disease, which only affects the skin, not systemic lupus. Ironically, she was disappointed by the news that she did not have systemic lupus erythematosus—her search for an "acceptable" explanation of her fatigue had come to an end. And her physician had failed to help her out of the morass.

Afternoon Exhaustion

My own attack of hepatitis vividly revealed to me what afternoon exhaustion was like. In my own case, I felt as if I were swimming against a strong tide, utterly exhausted by an effort that was getting me nowhere. By 2:00 in the afternoon, the most ordinary task defeated me. Working was out of the question.

Very little is known about this type of fatigue. The late German writer Thomas Mann described it in detail in his novel *The Magic Mountain,* with its brilliant cast of characters taking "the cure" in an Alpine tuberculosis sanitarium. For all practical purposes, this form of fatigue is virtually always due to a medical illness, such as infection, inflammation, or tumor. The associated disease may not be a serious one: Think of the flu that gets you down for a week. Unlike early morning lassitude, rest can ameliorate this type of fatigue; this is why the patient with fatigue related to a medical disease tends to feel best after a restful night's sleep.

CAUSES OF FATIGUE

Inflammation is a response the body uses as a defense against invading microbes. In an autoimmune disease like systemic lupus erythematosus, the body suffers from attack by the very inflammatory mechanisms that it musters as an antimicrobial defense. One result of this is the production of small proteins of the immune system termed lymphokines, which signal other cells to carry out particular functions.

An extremely important lymphokine is interleukin-1, discovered by Dr. Charles Dinarello and Dr. Sheldon Wolff, of the New England Medical Center and the Tufts University School of Medicine. Interleukin-1, or IL-1, has many different effects on the body. Two of its important activities concern its ability to stimulate certain cells in the brain. Cells in the part of the brain called the hypothalamus respond to IL-1 by causing a rise in the body's temperature: fever. Other brain cells respond to IL-1 by producing yet another peptide that causes sleep. Injection of highly purified IL-1 will put a rabbit to sleep. Another lymphokine, TNF, has the same sleep-inducing property.

Equally interesting is that substances in certain bacteria will themselves induce sleep; so a person infected with, say, *tuberculosis bacilli* will feel tired for at least two reasons: the body's own sleep-inducing lymphokines and those contained in the microbe itself.

Fever and rest (sleep) are part of the defense against infection. They are imposed on the patient by the body's response to the infection, which includes the production of specific fever-inducing and sleep-inducing peptide messengers. Your mother was right when she told you to go to bed when you had a bad cold! What remains to be shown is that these same mechanisms occur in the patient with active systemic lupus erythematosus—presumably they do, but actual evidence is lacking. If it is indeed true that IL-1 and TNF induce fatigue in lupus, then physicians would have at their disposal an objective means of evaluating and advising the vexed, tired lupus patient.

PART FIVE

Lupus: Its Diagnosis and Medications Used to Treat It

27

Did Medications Trigger My Disease or Spur My Recovery?

by Henrietta Aladjem

Since early childhood, I have shown a sensitivity to medications. Many drugs that help other people, instead of helping me, caused problems that were never interpreted correctly. These reactions could and should have been a warning signal from nature. Yet for nearly twenty years, I passively swallowed pills and took injections without thinking twice. I should have learned from experience, but I had to be hit over the head with these reactions many, many times before reaching the right conclusions. Now I think twice before I even take aspirin.

When I had active lupus, I took large doses of cortisone, which caused fluid retention. To alleviate the resulting discomfort, I took diuretics. For pains and aches I took aspirin—as many as sixteen each day. For stomach distress, I took atropine, pyrabenzamine, Gelusil, and other drugs. For a chronic sore throat, I took small doses of penicillin and tetracycline. (It was later determined that I was sensitive to both.) I also took potassium chloride, vitamins B_6 and B_{12}, ascorbic acid, and folic acid. Along with these vitamins and drugs, my doctors instituted niacin injections (vitamin B_3, 1 cc per day), autogenous vaccines made from my own bacteria, and white cell injections (5 cc each time).

The white cell injections were recommended by a rheumatologist from California who came all the way to Boston to consult on my case. He believed that patients with SLE could benefit from these injections and gave them to all his patients indefinitely. However, the treatment was not proven scientifically, and he had no idea how the injections worked. He based his theory on the premise that some enzyme caused damage to the DNA, and normal white cells supplied the missing factor, thus inhibiting the damage. From the conversation by my bedside, I learned that the California physician worked at a Los Angeles hospital with 3,500 beds, where he had an LE research laboratory. In that laboratory, several thousand such white cell treatments had been performed on patients. The California physician mentioned that in several other hospitals in the country, tests were randomly performed on all patients with SLE or where other rheumatic diseases were suspected. At one point, the physicians standing by my bedside laughed when one of them suggested, jokingly, that the white blood cell injections be given to all women with diagnostic problems. Before the California doctor left, he advised a regimen of increased doses of cortisone, plus the white blood cell injections twice a week. These injections were bearable only because I hoped for their success.

Years later, when I served on the National Advisory Council at N.I.A.I.D., at the National Institute of Health in Bethesda, Maryland, there was one council member who had been an intern at Peter Bent Brigham Hospital when I was a patient there. We recalled that he had given me the white blood cell injections when my own rheumatologist, Dr. Gardner, was not available. At a council meeting, he spoke about the white blood cell injections and explained that they had the potential to cause a severe, even lethal, immune reaction.

The doctor had a sheepish glimmer in his eyes when he said that he hoped I would not remember that he had given me the white cell injections. I had no comment; however, I was thinking that I was lucky to be alive. I had taken those injections for a whole year. When Dr. Gardner gave me the hundredth injection, he decided to stop them. He reasoned that by the law of averages, chances were that I could get infected with hepatitis. I tried not to think about that!

Dr. Gardner was willing to try anything to help me. He gave me large doses of cortisone right after the diagnosis, hoping to quickly bring about a remission. He relied on his medical education, his trained intuition, my medical history, and other factors. Recently, a group of Dutch scientists published a paper[1] entitled, "Prevention of Relapses in Systemic Lupus Erythematosus" (Jarman, P., P. Bootsma, et al. *Lancet* June 24, 1995 345: 1595–1599). The study is promising. If this work is proven successful, Dr. Gardner's experiment might have been, at least in part, responsible for my remission.

In 1953, physicians knew little about the toxicity or side effects of steroids. They had no idea why antimalarial drugs worked, or even why aspirin alleviated pain or helped inflammation. Patients had to accept the immediate side effects of these drugs, as well as the long-term side effects that might not occur until years later.

The list of experimental drugs used to treat lupus is still frightening, and which drugs are prescribed depends on which research center you go to and who the attending physician there is.

My Bulgarian physician, Dr. Liuben Popoff, whom I met in Leon, France, some years ago, believed that every drug will find the patient who reacts badly to it. "Even so," he said, "every time I see a drug reaction, I think of lupus." He added that many people have a quiet form of lupus or a predisposition to the disease, and doctors bring out the illness by giving them too many medications for innocent complaints. "The medications lead to new complaints," he said, "and we chase the problem with new medications. Often, we believe that the patient is neurotic. The neurosis starts and finishes our chase. It is difficult to tell for sure in some patients."

Even though adverse drug effects can occur, as we will see in Neil Duane's case in a later article, physicians seem to accept these side effects as inevitable—a necessary evil. While talking to Neil Duane, I wondered when physicians would become more willing to understand and less willing to prescribe.

28

Lupus and Medications

by Henrietta Aladjem
in Conversation With Stephen R. Kaplan, M.D., F.A.C.P.

A few years ago, when Dr. Stephen Kaplan was Professor of Medicine at Brown University Medical School and Chief of Rheumatology at Roger Williams Hospital in Providence, I interviewed him about lupus and medications for a previous book of mine *Understanding Lupus*. Today, his submission still stands, and with a few minor revisions, it is reprinted in this book.

Dr. Kaplan addressed several general issues before discussing some of the specific characteristics of the drugs that are used in the treatment of lupus. He pointed out that many manifestations of systemic lupus erythematosus (SLE) are treatable. Some medications affect the mechanisms of the disease in ways that alter lupus' signs and symptoms. Many of these therapeutic agents actually treat the disease process and should not be considered just symptomatic treatment.

"Unfortunately," he said, "among those patients whose involvement with SLE affects their kidneys or central nervous system, there are some whose disease will not be affected or controlled by currently available medical means. In dealing with these severe problems, we reach the frontiers of modern therapeutics, and when faced with such critical medical circumstances, we must carefully judge the point at which the chances of helping the individual with the aggressive use of potent medications become outweighed by the chance of doing them harm. These considerations of 'doing no harm,' even in extreme situations, have taken on added significance as we appreciate that improvement, such as in the supportive care of patients with central nervous system disease, may provide a critical period of time in which some spontaneous improvement may occur. In patients with the severest forms of renal disease, medicine is now capable of providing kidney dialysis or even kidney transplantation."

Dr. Kaplan stressed that no cure for lupus is known at this time. However, he says, curability is not always a simple concept; many serious illnesses, such as diabetes or some forms of heart disease, may not be curable today but can frequently be controlled sufficiently to permit a normal lifestyle. Treatability, therefore, should be emphasized in disorders like SLE, so that patients and their physicians can work toward realistic expectations, and not feel unnecessarily tormented or driven by overly optimistic or pessimistic notions. Dr. Kaplan believes that any treatment program should include the intelligent use of preventive measures by the patient, such as appropriate protection from the sun when photosensitivity is a problem and from temperature extremes when Raynaud's phenomenon (spasm of the arteries of the fingers resulting in poor circulation) is present.

Drugs, however, play a critical role in dealing with the treatable manifestations of SLE. Without doubt, most medications that are used in lupus and other serious medical problems are double-edged swords. Their potential to produce significant benefit must be considered in balance with their potential for producing adverse effects and added problems for the patients. We are all aware of the great feats a skilled mechanic can perform in repairing complex machinery with the proper tools; in contrast, we can also imagine the harm that can be done with the same tools, including the proverbial monkey wrench, when applied improperly or carelessly. In medical therapeutics, medications are highly specialized tools with the capacity to alter complex reactions in a way that benefits the patient.

Dr. Kaplan said, "Patients need to maintain a level of prescribed medications sufficient to affect the mechanisms of SLE. Since the body is continually inactivating and eliminating the drugs, maintaining a desirable effect by a drug depends on cooperation by the patient. Taking the medication so that the effect is fairly continuous prevents SLE from returning or gaining the upper hand. This must be balanced, of course, by the potential for each drug to produce adverse side effects. One must keep the potential for these side effects in proper perspective. The principle in selecting the medication and dose should be in keeping with a sentiment expressed in Gilbert and Sullivan's *Mikado:* 'Let the [potential] punishment fit the crime.' Clearly, all patients should be knowledgeable about the medications they administer to themselves. If a side effect does appear, changing the dosage or shifting to an equivalent but different medication should follow deliberation involving both patient and physician."

Before discussing which medications are used in the treatment of lupus, it is important to understand that every medication has three names. Each drug has a chemical name that is generally not well known except to chemists working in the laboratory. Each drug is also given a generic name, which is a shorthand for the complicated chemical name. This generic name is used to refer to a specific medication, regardless of manufacturer. The third name for each drug is the trade name, which is the name a manufacturer uses to identify its proprietary product. Some states mandate that if a drug is prescribed by its trade name, the least expensive generic equivalent carried by the pharmacy must be used to fill the prescription. All drugs in this chapter will be referred to by their generic names with some trade names following in parentheses.

CORTICOSTEROIDS

Many lupus patients take various forms of corticosteroids, and some experience adverse effects from long-term regular usage. There are now drugs available to replace cortisone. According to Dr. Kaplan, after cortisone and its properties were discovered, many different forms of this drug were created in the laboratory, such as prednisone, prednisolone, triamcinolone, and others. These drugs are generally stronger than the original chemical, but all have the same adverse effects. These drugs, which physicians refer to as steroids or corticosteroids, are among the most potent drugs known to suppress inflammation. Steroids may also suppress the activity of the immune system. In lupus, a disturbance in the immune system regulation results in the inappropriate inflammatory activity responsible for many of the signs and symptoms of lupus. The powerful *anti*-inflammatory effect of steroids may be used in various manners to manage lupus.

Steroid creams can control lupus skin rashes, as well as nose ulcers. Such creams can often prevent the serious scarring that once characterized the progression of these SLE manifestations. Prolonged use of some of the newer and more powerful steroid creams may cause injury to the skin, so patients should discuss the situation with their physicians who recommend prolonged use of this topical medication.

Some steroid preparations may be injected directly into a joint affected by SLE arthritis, says Dr. Kaplan, when arthritis remains active in spite of other measures. Physicians worry about harming a patient with steroid therapy, not so much with its topical or intra-articular (within the joint) use, as when the medication is administered on a regular basis over a long period of time.

I asked Dr. Kaplan to explain what cortisone compounds are.

"There are hormones that are normally produced by the adrenal gland in each of us every day. Most of the time a fairly constant amount is produced each day, but when placed under stress, our bodies require increased amounts of these materials to maintain the metabolism that supports blood pressure, maintains a normal balance of chemicals in the blood, and so on. A primary control for the amount of cortisone the adrenal glands produce is another hormone called adrenocorticotropic hormone (ACTH), which is produced by the pituitary gland at the base of the skull. One way to produce increased amounts of cortisone, therefore, is to administer increased amounts of ACTH by injection. This is a simple substitute for the administration of steroids, but it has little or no particular advantage over the more easily administered steroid pills.

"Cortisone is an important part of the metabolic systems in our body, and affects the stores of body sugar, protein, and fats, thereby helping to maintain an adequate supply and balance of these nutrients. Cortisone also affects the balance of chemicals in the blood that are important in maintaining normal blood pressure and hydration. Although many of these side effects are not dependent on exactly the same actions as the anti-inflammatory effects of the steroids, the anti-inflammatory activity system has not yet been isolated from the activity of the metabolic systems, with many consequences for the patient. Thus, steroid use should be thoroughly discussed by the patient and physician."

Flannery O'Conner, the Southern author who died from lupus in 1964, wrote that when she was on steroids, her face became round like a watermelon. There was a time when I looked like that myself. Dr. Kaplan explained that the impact of steroids on the metabolic system may include redistribution of the fatty stores of the body, causing the face to become round—the so-called "moon face." Steroids can also raise blood sugar above normal, increase appetite (which may result in weight gain), cause some weakening of the bony structures because of interference with calcium metabolism, increase the risk of developing infections, produce cataracts, etc. Many people, however, do take therapeutically beneficial amounts of steroids and experience relatively few of these many potential adverse effects.

Physicians planning to prescribe steroids should develop a clear list of problems for which they are seeking solutions so that, when the treatment is started, an objective analysis of its success can be made and weighed against the risks of the treatment. It's important to perform this evaluation, according to Dr. Kaplan, because individuals vary in their ability to tolerate the same doses of steroid medication. The patient can only be a cooperating partner if he or she appreciates the benefits of the treatment objectively as well as subjectively. This understanding also helps put the activity of a disease like lupus in perspective. Steroid therapy must be gradually reduced once it has produced satisfactory results, but the physician's effort must be to maintain the beneficial effects while reducing the chance of adverse effects. As many know, this is often a difficult, as well as delicate, task.

Children with lupus face some additional problems with this treatment, since steroids may affect their growth rate. When an individual is receiving steroids, the normal activity of the adrenal gland—to make cortisone in response to ACTH stimulation—is suppressed and dulled. This dovetails with the *other* major reason why an individual who has been receiving steroids for a prolonged period of time must reduce the dose gradually. According to Dr. Kaplan, gradually reducing the dose will permit the adrenal gland to regain its sensitivity to ACTH, particularly with the lower doses of steroids.

How long can patients safely take steroids? Dr. Kaplan stresses that one way to retain many of the beneficial effects of steroids and reduce some of their unwanted adverse effects is to provide the treatment over the briefest possible period. As long as their therapeutic benefits can be maintained, the steroids should be taken at one time in the morning, rather than spaced out over the day, and taken only every other day. Again, this should be done only with careful and specific directions from a physician, and only as long as the therapy's usefulness is retained. Occasionally, however, a physician may decide to eliminate steroids altogether after a very prolonged period of excellent control of the disease, sometimes several months. This requires an extremely close working relationship between physician and patient, since careful judgments must be made about how to treat any minor symptoms that appear, not as manifestations of SLE, but as a result of the reduced steroid intake.

In summary, Dr. Kaplan thinks that steroid therapy is the epitome of the double-edged sword image of medical treatment, even when it is life-saving. It should be used for those manifestations of lupus that must be controlled and that cannot be treated adequately by other, less potent means. Clinical researchers are trying to document the circumstances when steroid therapy is most helpful and appropriate and develop newer compounds that will fight inflammation effects without the dangerous side effects. In recent years, investigators have tried to develop new dosage regimens that produce fewer side effects. One dosage regimen in current use is called "pulse therapy," in which very large single doses of steroids are administered intravenously for three consecutive days. This type of program is considered most often when the patient's condition appears to be deteriorating despite significant daily doses of steroids and/or other SLE medications. While pulse therapy does seem to reduce the long-term adverse effects of steroids, such as the loss of calcium from bone and the redistribution of the fatty tissues, it is not totally free of associated problems. Following such therapy with corticosteroids, some patients have developed seizures or serious bacterial infections.

NONSTEROIDAL ANTI-INFLAMMATORY DRUGS (NSAIDS)

One group of widely used drugs that suppress inflammation is unrelated to any form of cortisone; these are referred to as nonsteroidal anti-inflammatory drugs (NSAIDs). NSAIDs can be further divided into smaller groups depending on their chemical structures. All these drugs are altered and gradually eliminated by chemical systems in the body, so that if a patient takes a medication only sporadically, the drug level required for an anti-inflammatory effect will not be reached and no improvement can be expected. This is an important difference, therefore, from just taking a couple of aspirin to alleviate an annoying pain or headache. It is also important to know that when anti-inflammatory doses of the NSAIDs are being used, increasing the dosage must be done very gradually, and the new blood level and improvement may not occur for four to five days after raising the dosage. NSAIDs have been used to treat some limited manifestations of inflammation in lupus, such as arthritis.

Aspirin does have side effects. According to Dr. Kaplan, some, but by no means all, patients with lupus who receive aspirin regularly may develop liver tissue changes that produce abnormalities in blood tests measuring liver health and function. For this reason, some physicians substitute other NSAIDs, which were developed primarily for use in other rheumatic disorders. Other, more generally known, adverse effects can result from treatment with aspirin, such as gastrointestinal distress. Occasionally, this distress can lead to an ulcer of the stomach wall. Minor gastrointestinal symptoms can sometimes be avoided by always taking aspirin right after meals with a large glass of water, and using special "buffered" coated aspirins that dissolve after passing through the stomach.

Most widely advertised over-the-counter preparations are mainly aspirin. Some aspirins whose names suggest they contain buffers do *not* have buffering strength sufficient to make a difference to those who must take large quantities of pills daily. Other widely advertised over-the-counter preparations that do not contain aspirin or any other salicylate usually contain acetaminophen (one example is Tylenol). Acetaminophen is less likely to irritate the stomach, but provides little or none of the anti-inflammatory activity that aspirin or other NSAIDs can.

Aspirin can also cause nervous system side effects. An early sign of this is a buzzing sound (called tinnitus) in the patient's ears. This harmless effect can be eliminated by decreasing the aspirin dose and thus avoiding the possibility of more serious side effects on the nervous system. Older individuals, who may lack the ability to hear this early warning sign, should receive special care and monitoring for signs of adverse effects, such as abrupt change in personality.

Aspirin also affects the normal functioning of the platelets, important components in blood clotting. Aspirin should be avoided when other drugs or SLE decrease the blood's ability to clot properly. However, low doses of aspirin (81 to 325 mg per day) may be given in some cases as a mild anticoagulant to prevent blood clotting.

In recent years, clinicians have also become aware of the potential of aspirin and other NSAIDs to affect kidney function. This is more likely to be a problem in people who suffer from diseases like SLE or diabetes that already affect the kidneys. When the kidneys are stressed by a systemic illness or inflammation, they become more dependent on their ability to make chemicals called prostaglandins, which help maintain proper blood flow to the kidneys. Aspirin and the other NSAIDs may block the ability to make prostaglandins and thus worsen kidney function. Although impaired kidney function does not occur frequently when lupus patients receive aspirin or other NSAIDs, kidney function should be monitored regularly and is of particular concern when a lupus flare-up occurs and the kidneys are stressed and/or inflamed.

Dr. Kaplan emphasizes that despite all these concerns, NSAIDs remain inexpensive and are potentially effective medications for dealing with some forms of inflammation in SLE. A dose of two aspirin, taken occasionally to alleviate a headache or a minor pain, is still one of the best bargains in health care.

Some new types of salicylates, such as choline magnesium trisalicylate (Trilisate) have been introduced into medical practice. According to Dr. Kaplan, these drugs are thought to produce fewer adverse stomach effects. Because these new NSAIDs stay in the bloodstream longer, the anti-inflammatory level can be maintained in the blood with lower doses or fewer pills. However, it is much more expensive than aspirin and can be obtained only by prescription, since the dose must be carefully controlled. At high levels, this drug may cause serious nervous system and metabolic side effects. High blood levels of salicylate are especially dangerous for children and the elderly, Dr. Kaplan emphasizes. People taking any salicylate regularly must be extremely careful to keep this medication away from children.

The second group of NSAIDs includes drugs such as indomethacin (Indocin) and medications of somewhat similar structure, tolmetin sodium (Tolectin) and sulindac (Clinoril). A third group of available NSAIDs includes three medications called ibuprofen (Motrin, Rufen), fenoprofen calcium (Nalfon), and naproxen (Naprosyn). Additional NSAIDs derived from other classes of similar kinds of compounds introduced into medical practice in recent years include meclofenamate sodium (Meclomen) and piroxicam (Feldene). Diflunisal (Dolobid) is also a relatively new NSAID; it is related to aspirin and was introduced primarily as a painkiller.

All the NSAIDs, in fact, have painkilling properties that are independent of their anti-inflammatory dose. In other words, if a person is already receiving one of these drugs for lupus inflammation at the appropriate dosage level, increasing the dosage is not likely to relieve further pain, but may increase the likelihood of an undesirable side effect. Also, if a patient is already taking a NSAID regularly for lupus and needs a pain pill for a dental extraction or some other reason, the additional pain pill should not be another NSAID. Any of these drugs might be used for minimal or moderate inflammation of the joints caused by SLE. Individuals vary widely in their response to these medications; it's hard to predict which will successfully control this inflammation and be well tolerated. Each medication must be taken regularly at a proper dose in order to maintain the desired level in the body. Remember, they are *never* interchangeable.

NSAIDs may work fairly rapidly compared with some other drugs, yet it may take three or four weeks before the full benefit is experienced. Several of the NSAIDs, including sulindac, naproxen, piroxicam, and diflunisal, normally stay longer in the body and, therefore, require fewer daily doses to have an anti-inflammatory effect. All these medications are relatively expensive, however, and this should be a consideration.

It is important to note that all these medications can cause gastrointestinal problems. Other possible adverse effects include mild dizziness and blurry vision. Indomethacin produces a high incidence of morning headaches, as well as a dulling of the senses and forgetfulness. Meclofenamate sodium can produce diarrhea. An adverse effect that has been specifically identified in lupus patients who take ibuprofen is occasional headache, malaise, and neck pain indicative of an aseptic meningitis (an *extremely* rare complication). If a patient is truly allergic to aspirin, experiences a hive-like rash (urticaria), or develops wheezing, he or she may have this same reaction when any other NSAID is prescribed. This seems more severe in patients who have a history of many allergies, and who have or have had nasal polyps. Kidneys that are inflamed or stressed because of systemic disease activity may become further impaired when the individual takes other NSAIDs besides aspirin. Any of these drugs may also cause fluid retention, as well as allergic reactions that may occur with any other medication. In fact, there is no extensive, well documented experience with any of these drugs in large numbers of SLE patients, although they are used with some success in selected clinical situations with the rheumatic manifestations of lupus.

According to Dr. Kaplan, the best source of information about the proper use of and precautions for all medications is "Dispensing Information—Advice for the Patient," published by the U.S. Pharmacopoeia, which calls on panels of experts to thoughtfully organize information about each drug for patients.

ANTIMALARIAL DRUGS

Hydroxychloroquine (Plaquenil), an altogether different type of medication, is also widely used in SLE treatment. It is related to a group of compounds first found to be useful in treating malaria, and then discovered to have unique anti-inflammatory properties. While other members of this family of drugs are occasionally used to treat SLE, hydroxychloroquine is the most widely prescribed. It has been found effective in controlling inflammation and, in particular, many of SLE skin manifestations.

Although it occurs rarely, according to Dr. Kaplan, one of the more serious adverse effects of antimalarial drugs is their tendency to accumulate in the retina of the eye, which may rarely result in blindness. This is clearly related to the total dose of the medication taken over time, so the recommended dose of this drug should not be exceeded. Deposits in the lens of the eye may also occur, and an early sign of that problem is when the patient complains about seeing halos around streetlights or lamps. These symptoms disappear when the drug is reduced or stopped. We must check frequently for potential problem of the drug accumulating in the retina. Other side effects may include gastrointestinal distress, skin rashes, and occasional muscle weakness or decreased hearing acuity. However, most individuals taking any one of these medications in proper and adequate doses do not experience any side effects. Hydroxychloroquine can be very effective in treating some problems in lupus patients, but it does take effect slowly. Improvement seldom occurs within one month, and three to six months may pass before the maximum benefit is noted.

CYTOTOXIC DRUGS

Some medications have been adopted for use in SLE not because of their potential to suppress inflammation directly, but because of their ability to affect the immune cells. A basic cause of the inflammation and injury to tissues and organs from SLE is a disturbance in the functioning of the immune system. Cytotoxic (cell-killing) drugs target this system.

According to Dr. Kaplan, medical researchers do not as yet understand all they need to know about the factors producing this kind of disturbance, although they are the object of a good deal of current research. "When drugs were developed to treat malignant diseases, they were designed to injure cells fatally, with the hope that the tumor cells would be more sensitive than the normal cells of the body. Researchers soon noted that certain cells of the immune system, the lymphocytes, were particularly susceptible to some of these medications, and the ability of the immune system to function was altered. When it was observed that these compounds might suppress immune system function, they were tested in patients with very severe forms of disorders like SLE, where the immune system appeared to be abnormal and contributing to the disease process. In patients who have undergone kidney transplantation, these drugs have proven necessary for satisfactory results.

Over the years, two cytotoxic drugs have been used with variable success both in patients with severe SLE unresponsive to other treatment and in those patients requiring unacceptably high doses of steroids. One of these drugs is azathioprine (Imuran), and the other is cyclophosphamide (Cytoxan, Neosan). The use of these drugs with SLE patients with serious kidney involvement remains one of the most discussed issues among rheumatologists. Some physicians think that these patients will tend to do at least as well by being on one of these medications, and lower doses of steroids, rather than on higher doses of steroids alone.

"While cytotoxic drugs do produce side effects, they are not the same effects produced by steroids; thus, the incidence and seriousness of the side effects from the overall treatment can be reduced using a combined approach. Because cytotoxic drugs can affect the normal, rapidly dividing cells in the bone marrow, the blood count of lupus patients taking them must be carefully monitored. As is true with all medications, and particularly with these drugs, the prescribing of drugs and the proper monitoring of the use should be a serious contractual arrangement between physician and patient. The patient not only has the right to be well informed about medications, but he or she must also understand and be committed to the monitoring procedures needed to make sure that the medication can be administered as safely as possible."

In addition to its effects on the blood count, azathioprine sometimes produces other adverse effects when it is first administered, including affecting the liver, or gastrointestinal distress. The dose may be reduced if an individual has pre-existing liver disease, or is taking a drug called allopurinal to reduce uric acid. In such cases, the dose of azathioprine must be very greatly reduced, and the patient's blood tests must be followed with great care. Cyclophosphamide, which some people feel may be preferable to azathioprine in similar circumstances, must also be given with extreme care and close monitoring. In addition to serious effects on the blood count and occasional gastrointestinal distress, regular usage may cause hair loss, although this is generally reversible. Another potential problem, according to Dr. Kaplan, is the tendency of the drug to produce bladder irritation; people with relatively normal kidney function who are taking cyclophosphamide are encouraged to drink ten to twelve extra glasses of water each day so that the irritating breakdown products of cyclophosphamide will not concentrate in the bladder.

Unfortunately, long-term complications with cyclophosphamide are possible. According to Dr. Kaplan, these include sterility, which may not be reversible. Cytotoxic drugs also have effects on DNA, the body's genetic material. Although normal babies have been delivered from parents taking drugs like azathioprine, physicians are concerned about the development *in utero* of a fetus conceived and maturing while a parent was taking one of those cytotoxic drugs. In addition, there is reason to believe that individuals taking these medications face an increased risk of developing certain malignancies later in life. While this risk has not been established for patients with SLE, information from other types of patients raise this as at least a theoretical possibility for the SLE patient receiving azathioprine or cyclophosphamide.

Because of these potential long-term effects and known short-term effects, cytotoxic drugs should be considered only in the severest form of lupus, or in an attempt to evade other unacceptable adverse effects from high doses of steroids. Advances in understanding of the metabolism of lymphocytes has recently led researchers to work toward the development of new types of agents that may manipulate the immune system in a manner more specific than is possible with currently available drugs. As we learn more about these drugs, we hope they will be looked at with regard to the serious problem of SLE.

29

Drug-Induced Lupus
Mimics Real S.L.E.

by Neil F. Duane

After giving a talk about the patients' perspective of lupus to the American Medical Writers Association in Boston, Neil F. Duane, former President of the Massachusetts Association, told me that after he was given medications for high blood pressure he developed a lupus-like disease. The disease disappeared after he stopped taking the medications. Sometime later, I interviewed Neil for Lupus Letter *and then later spoke with him again and asked him to revise his story for this book.*

Neil is a likable man in his late forties, with a ruddy complexion and lively, intelligent eyes. He appears full of drive and energy—not at all like someone who has had to put up with such serious medical problems—like having a kidney transplant.

Here is Neil's revised and updated version about his induced type of lupus:

Hydralazine, a commonly prescribed drug to control high blood pressure, and marketed under the trade name Apresoline, is only one of about two dozen drugs capable of producing a syndrome indistinguishable from systemic lupus erythematosus (SLE). The list of SLE-inducing prescription medicine includes birth control pills, as well as antibiotics, such as penicillin, streptomycin, and the tetracyclines, among others. In cases of those taking hydralazine, SLE can develop in approximately 10 percent of patients taking more than 200 milligrams per day. Other studies indicate that as many as one-fifth of persons taking over 200 milligrams a day may be susceptible.

Twenty-three years ago, I was a physically active 32-year-old white male with high blood pressure (180/110) secondary to polycystic kidney disease, a congenital condition unlikely to cause trouble until the fifth decade of life. Outwardly, I was healthy (kidney function still normal, no detectable cardiovascular impairment). But left untreated, this blood pressure exposed me to the unacceptable risks of developing heart disease, stroke, or "end-organ damage" to the still-functioning kidneys. The antihypertensive therapy my doctor prescribed included hydralazine, along with a diuretic, and eventually propranolol, (Inderal) a drug classified as a beta blocker, which helps reduce blood pressure by reducing cardiac output.

Antihypertensive drugs are often prescribed in combinations such as this because the actions of one drug often complement another taken at the same time. Sometimes the added drug will offset undesirable side effects of the others, and dozens of undesirable side effects are not uncommon. Since I was taking 400 mg of hydralazine a day, my odds of developing SLE were one in five to one in ten.

The first sign that I had developed hydralazine-induced lupus was early-morning stiffness in the finger and metacarpal (the bone that connects the knuckle joint of my little finger to the wrist) joints of my left hand. The stiffness was accompanied by the dull, persistent ache of what could only be described as "arthritic."

The onset and progression of the disease was insidious. As a regular cross-country skier and runner, I was used to aches and pains caused by wrenched knees, sprained wrists, and whacked elbows, so occasional stiffness and discomfort was more or less normal—the price one paid for "fitness."

In the early stages of my lupus, I was able to ignore it. Upon arising in the morning, the stiffness was quite pronounced, but as the day wore on and my circulation improved through normal exercise, the symptoms abated somewhat, and I was able to get through the day without undue discomfort.

Over a period of about two weeks or so, perhaps longer, I developed a noticeable limp caused by stiffness in my left knee and hip, especially when I arose from my desk to visit the engineering lab, or to get a cup of coffee. I worked the stiffness out as I walked. It wasn't until another technical writer Ralph Greenidge, who also ran track in his youth and was the father of three teenaged athletes, taunted me by cheerfully asking one morning if I had "clipped the last hurdle," did I think there was a problem.

Although we whistled past the graveyard together about the ravages of advancing age, privately I became concerned. Some would say it was about time. The disease progressed. More joints—the ankles and hips—stiffened, not only in the mornings but after periods of relatively short inactivity at the computer terminal, and after driving short distances.

I became listless, and I tired more easily. While working to install a new wooden deck on my house, I found that I could not grip a hammer well enough to drive a nail. Yet I persevered, clumsily missing the nails, and frequently dropping the hammer. At one point, I went so far as to lash the hammer to my hand with strips of duct tape, before finally surrendering the hammer to a helper. My knees grew worse, and I soon found it difficult to rise without support. I had become, for all intents and purposes, legally handicapped.

In retrospect, I have to wonder why I did not immediately see that something was seriously amiss. Why did I feel that if I just rested for awhile, I'd feel better? Why did I think that I was only experiencing the normal aches and pains that come when you enter the third decade of life? I think perhaps, that having never experienced serious disease, I didn't know what to expect, and therefore tried subconsciously to "will" it away.

Since my discomfort didn't appear to be life threatening, I assumed that my condition would either get better, or stay more or less the same, which I would live with. A month passed. It wasn't all steady decline. I'd have good days, and bad days. I continued to take my hydralazine, and my blood pressure was responding to the treatment.

At my next visit to the doctor, he asked the routine examination question of whether or not I had any pains in the joints. My answer this time was "yes"—not an emphatic "yes," but a non-complaining tentative "yes, but only in the mornings," I rationalized, "and not a lot of pain," or words to that effect.

A month later, the "yes" was no longer tentative. The arthritis-like stiffness was worse, and I had developed a rash on my face around my nose and eyes. "I think I might have hydralazine-induced lupus," I told my doctor. I worked for a medical electronics manufacturer and had access to an excellent medical library. I reviewed the "indications and contraindications" leaflets packaged with the hydralazine, and the long list of potential side effects in the *Physician's Desk Reference* (PDR). This wasn't a possibility to be lightly dismissed, and it occurred to me that given the symptoms, my doctor, an internist, was not inclined to take chances, however remote the possibility.

"If you like, we can order some blood work and check to see if you might have lupus," he said, making it sound like my decision. I decided that we'd run the test.

Three days later my doctor was on the phone. "Stop taking the hydralazine. Your tests are positive. You were right." I had the answer that I somehow knew already. I stopped taking hydralazine. My SLE-like symptoms improved, and the tests reverted to normal. Fortunately, in drug-induced lupus such as mine, there is a lower incidence of kidney involvement, anemia, and luekopenia than in spontaneous SLE, the nondrug-induced form of the disease. I got well far more quickly than I became ill. Recovery wasn't insidious; it was close to miraculous in its speed.

Suppose, I asked my doctor, almost insanely, I kept taking the hydralazine? What would happen? Would I develop full-blown lupus, light sensitivity, and all the other symptoms of the disease? "I don't know, and we don't want to find out," was his eminently sensible answer, completely devoid of scientific curiosity—end of scholarly debate. I didn't want to seriously pursue the possibilities either.

Still, I can't help but think, if the condition is reversible when the hydralazine is withdrawn, can something be learned that could benefit those who have a progressive form of the disease? Could drug-induced lupus patients serve a similar role? Having experienced lupus, I'd need to think hard about this—voluntarily inducing the lupus again.

Questions remain. Why did the stiffness occur on the left side? Was it because of old injuries that made these joints more susceptible? I know of no studies or research utilizing drug-induced lupus patients, other than those performed by the drug manufacturers during clinical trials, and these are only to discover potential side effects.

I recovered completely. Follow-up tests revealed no LE cells. No aches, no pains. My blood pressure is now being controlled with another drug, diet, and exercise. After recovering from my brush with lupus, I ran twelve miles a week; I ran on the beach, and in the sun and through the surf. I bought new cross-country skis and took my first alpine skiing lessons. No arthritic symptoms, except for a twinge in the right knee from the skiing lesson, not, I prayed, the lupus returning.

Since then my blood pressure has been controlled effectively (140/90) with a combination of Cardizem CD and propranolol, with no recurrence of lupus. My congenital kidney disease, however, gradually progressed as expected, until I was forced to begin hemodialysis in February of 1996, at the age of 55.

In June of 1996, I was extremely fortunate to receive a kidney transplant, a near-perfect match, which has allowed me to function normally without dialysis. I experienced one acute rejection episode, which was controlled aggressively with the immunosuppressant drug OKT3. I am now taking daily doses of cyclosporine (Neoral), prednisone, and CellCept (mycophenolate mofetil) to control rejection.

During the work day, I seldom think about lupus, unless the subject comes up in conversation (not often). But I still flex my fingers and toes every morning, testing for stiffness and pain, and feel a special empathy with everyone still meeting a new day with the solitary challenge of lupus.

30

Critique of Neil Duane's Story

by Malcolm P. Rogers, M.D.

After reading Neil Duane's story, Dr. Malcolm Rogers wrote:

First, I am struck by how knowledgeable this patient became about the phenomenon of drug-induced lupus; although it is not surprising, given his background as a medical writer. Furthermore, he had been dealing with his own medical problems from an early age: high blood pressure, linked to polycystic kidney disease. It serves as a reminder for us as physicians that the more aware we are of the backgrounds of our patients, the better we can understand their response to illness.

For me, the ultimate lesson in this story is that it is important to provide enough information to patients to allow them to fully participate in their own care. In this case, information about the risks of hydralazine would have allowed Mr. Duane to better interpret the symptoms he experienced. One wonders why every patient taking large doses of hydralazine, whose odds of developing SLE are reportedly between 10 percent and 20 percent, would not automatically be warned of the possibility of hydralazine-induced lupus.

This is also a classic story of the way in which we develop explanations of symptoms for ourselves. Generally, we attempt to explain them with the most benign or ordinary explanation, such as "over-exercise" or minor muscle pulls. For the most of us, minor strains and injuries do account for most of our musculoskeletal symptoms.

The other classic process presented by Mr. Duane is the use of denial. It is psychologically adaptive for most of us to remain optimistic and to put the best spin on different circumstances. He carried this to an extreme, at one point "lashing the hammer to his hand with strips of duct tape before finally surrendering the hammer to a helper." He didn't want to see himself as seriously ill, and he didn't want to give up activities. We all have an enormous drive to function and maintain meaningful activities in our lives. We do not wish to give in to symptoms, and often feel empowered to will ourselves to do things in spite of symptoms.

Mr. Duane denied the importance of his symptoms as long as he could. Comments of friends would occasionally break through his denial. Finally, when he developed a rash on his face and nose, he was driven to investigate this himself. He himself made the initial diagnosis and pushed his physician into checking it out.

His account goes on to describe a miraculously rapid recovery, once he stopped taking the hydralazine.

He raises some very interesting questions about the biology of drug-induced lupus, specifically, what would have happened had he continued taking the hydralazine. He seems disappointed by the lack of scientific curiosity in the response of his physician. Mr. Duane might have hoped for more collegial interaction between him and his physician, in which they would share not only the enormous enthusiasm for his recovery, but the distress of symptoms and even an intellectual and scientific curiosity about the disease that afflicted him. The patient pursued his own curiosity by describing his own experience and posing a series of questions. These kinds of questions are, in fact, exactly what leads to scientific advances. For example, what could be learned about lupus from the fact that this medication can trigger the disease? Why did stiffness first occur on one side? Was there some interaction between a previous injury process and hydralazine?

Later on, the progression of his polycystic kidney disease required a kidney transplant and immunosuppressant therapy. Perhaps he wondered whether or not those treatments would have been beneficial to lupus had that condition continued. Most of us are interested and acute observers of our own bodies and the investigators of the human condition. Some of the most helpful scientific questions and ideas may, in fact, come from our patients.

One also wonders what impact a serious and potentially life-threatening illness such as drug-induced lupus might have. The threat of such a serious illness undoubtedly also contributed to the strength of his initial denial. Denial is a way of limiting the psychological impact at the time, and keeping ourselves from residual sense of vulnerability after a serious illness, even after the disease has gone into remission. They also may gain greater appreciation for the fragility of life, and sometimes gain great appreciation for the pleasures of living in the moment.

31

Some Thoughts Related to Lupus and Medications

by Peter H. Schur, M.D.

SOME GENERAL RECOMMENDATIONS

The following are some general recommendations that should be followed in addition to taking any prescribed drugs for the control of one's lupus.

Diet and Nutrition

Limited data exist concerning the effect of dietary modification in SLE. One study reported that frequent eating of meat was associated with more active and progressive disease. In contrast, dietary fish oil has been reported to be beneficial. One double-blind, randomized study found that fourteen of seventeen patients who ingested 20 grams per day of eicosapentaeoic acid, an active component of fish oil, achieved either a useful or ideal status; in contrast thirteen of seventeen receiving placebo (a dummy drug) were worse or had not changed. These findings await confirmation; at present, we do not recommend fish oil supplements in the treatment of SLE.

A conservative approach is to recommend a balanced diet consisting of carbohydrates, proteins, and fats. However, the diet should be modified based upon disease activity and the response to therapy. Patients with active inflammatory disease and fever may require an increase in caloric intake.

Steroids enhance appetite, resulting in potentially significant weight gain. Hunger can be somewhat lessened by the ingestion of water, antacids, and/or H2 blockers. If, however, weight gain is significant, patients should receive information on low-calorie diets.

Significant hyperlipidemia (excessive fat in the bloodstream) may be induced by nephrotic syndrome or the administration of steroids. One study, for example, found that increasing one's prednisone dose by 10 milligrams per day was associated with an elevation in serum cholesterol of 7.5 milligrams per deciliter (0.2 millimoles per liter).

Patients with hyperlipidemia should be encouraged to eat a low-fat diet. A lipid-lowering agent (usually a statin) should be considered if cholesterol levels remain high despite a change in diet. Vitamins are rarely needed when patients eat a balanced diet. However, a daily multivitamin should be taken by patients who are not able to find or afford healthy food, or who are dieting to lose weight. Patients on long-term steroids and postmenopausal women should also ingest 400 to 800 international units of vitamin D plus 1,000 milligrams of calcium per day to minimize bone loss.

Exercise

Inactivity produced by acute illness causes a rapid loss of muscle mass and stamina. Fatigue may, therefore, ensue, even after the illness subsides. This can usually be treated with graded exercise. In selected refractory (resistant to treatment) cases, relief of fatigue can be obtained with prednisone or dehydroepiandrosterone (DHEA), a hormone.

Immunizations

It had been previously thought that immunization could exacerbate SLE. However, the influenza vaccine has now been shown to be safe and effective; the pneumococcal vaccine is also safe, but resultant antibody levels are somewhat lower in patients with SLE than in people without the disease. Keep in mind, however, that it is inadvisable to immunize patients receiving steroids or cytotoxic therapy with live vaccines, because these drugs cause immune suppression that may promote infection.

Avoidance of Specific Medications

Anecdotal data suggest that sulfonamides and penicillin (but not the synthetic penicillins) may exacerbate lupus and should, therefore, be avoided. In contrast, medications that cause drug-induced lupus, such as procainamide and hydralazine, do *not* exacerbate idiopathic SLE. This observation is thought to reflect pathogenetic differences between the two disorders.

Contraceptives

Oral contraceptives containing high doses of estrogen can exacerbate SLE. However, this complication rarely occurs with the current crop of low-dose estrogen- or progesterone-containing compounds. Patients with migraine headaches, Raynaud's syndrome, a history of phlebitis, or antiphospholipid antibodies probably should not be treated with oral contraceptives. We also recommend avoidance of intrauterine devices, due to the increased risk of infection.

TREATMENT OF BLOOD DISORDERS

The anemia of chronic inflammation in SLE usually responds to high-dose corticosteroids (1 milligram per kilogram per day of prednisone or its equivalent in divided doses). Immunosuppressive agents also may help, but at the transient risk of further bone marrow suppression. Bone marrow suppression can also be induced by medications, including antimalarials and immunosuppressive drugs.

Hemolytic Anemia

Hemolytic anemia, characterized by an elevated reticulocyte (the youngest red blood cells) count, *low* haptoglobin (a protein constituent of the blood) levels, and a positive direct Coombs test has been noted in 10 to 40 percent of patients with SLE. Currently, the incidence of hemolytic anemia is at the lower end of the above range, presumably due to earlier and better SLE therapy. Other patients have a positive Coombs test without evidence of overt hemolysis. The presence of both immunoglobulin and complement on the red cell is usually associated with some degree of hemolysis, while the presence of complement alone (e.g., C3 and/or C4) is often not associated with hemolysis. The antibodies are "warm," IgG, and are directed against Rh determinants. IgM mediated cold agglutinin hemolysis is uncommon.

Hemolytic anemia responds to steroids (1 milligram per killigram per day of prednisone or its equivalent in divided doses) in approximately 75 percent of patients. Once the hematocrit (the volume percentage of red blood cells in the blood) begins to rise and the reticulocyte count falls, steroids can be rapidly tapered. If there is no response, one can consider pulse steroids, immunosuppressant agents like azathioprine (up to 2 mg/kg per day) and cyclophosphamide (up to 2 milligrams per kilogram), or surgical removal of the spleen. Success rates for splenectomy (removal of the spleen) as high as 60 percent have been reported, although others have found no benefit. Other anecdotally described approaches to patients with refractory disease include intravenous immune globulin and danazol (in doses of 600 to 800 milligrams per day).

Leukopenia

Leukopenia in SLE rarely requires treatment, with the exception of patients with concurrent fever thought to be due to lupus or those with recurrent infections. In the latter setting, steroids (e.g., prednisone at 10 to 60 milligrams per day) may raise the white blood cell count and thereby help fight the infection. However, although prednisone or immunosuppressive agents (e.g., azathioprine and cyclophosphamide) can raise the white blood cell count, they can also result in an increased risk of infections and/or worsening of the leukopenia via bone marrow suppression.

Thrombocytopenia

Platelet counts of less than 50,000 per milliliter rarely cause more than prolonged bleeding time, while counts of less than 20,000 per milliliter may be associated with (and account for) petechia, purpura, ecchymoses, epistaxis, gingival, and other clinical bleeding. Treatment of thrombocytopenia is usually recommended for symptomatic patients with platelet counts lower than 50,000 per milliliter and for all patients with counts lower than 20,000 per milliliter.

The treatment of idiopathic thrombocytopenic purpura in SLE is the same as that in patients without lupus. Reviewed briefly, the mainstay of treatment is prednisone 1 mg per kilogram per day in divided doses. Most patients respond within one to eight weeks. If there is no significant increase in the platelet count within one to three weeks or side effects are intolerable, several options may be considered. The order in which they are used depends in part upon the severity of the thrombocytopenia and the presence or absence of other manifestations of SLE. Some of these options include:

- Azathioprine (0.5 mg/kg per day).

- Cyclophosphamide, given as daily oral or intravenous pulse therapy. Intravenous pulse cyclophosphamide is preferred in patients who have severe active lupus nephritis. In one report of six such patients, all had normal platelet counts within two to eighteen weeks after the onset of pulse cyclophosphamide.

- Intravenous immune globulin is very effective and may be preferred to azathioprine or cyclophosphamide when a rapid rise in platelet count is necessary (as in the patient who is actively bleeding or requires emergent surgery).

- Splenectomy, which should be preceded by immunization with pneumococcal vaccine prior to splenectomy. Although splenectomy can raise the platelet count, it does not cure the disease, as relapse is common, occurring up to fifty-four months after surgery.

- Danazol (400 to 800 mg/day). In one report, six of six patients who were unresponsive to other therapies responded to danazol (200 mg four times a day) within six weeks; this benefit occurred without a change in platelet-bound IgG antibodies. The dose could be tapered without relapse in five of the six patients.

- Vincristine.

TREATMENT OF PAIN

Multiple drugs are available to treat the pain syndromes of SLE. Nonsteroidal antiinflammatory drugs (NSAIDs) or acetaminophen are typically used first since the arthralgia and arthritis of SLE generally respond to these medications. Other drugs are added if necessary.

- If inflammation (swelling, redness, warmth) is the most prominent feature, we favor NSAIDs over full-dose aspirin (which requires too many pills). A typical dose of ibuprofen is 800 mg four times a day, of naproxen is 500 mg twice a day, and of nabumetone is 500 mg four times a day.

- If patients are complaining mostly of pain, we favor acetaminophen (up to 4 g/day in the absence of liver disease or alcoholism).

- Antimalarial drugs (e.g., hydroxychloroquine 200 to 400 mg/day) are very effective for the amelioration of joint symptoms and prevention of clinical relapse. Hydroxychloroquine (Plaquenil) is typically given to patients with articular manifestations (usually added to an NSAID in a nonresponder), rashes, and fatigue.

- Dehydroepiandrosterone (DHEA) (200 mg/day) has shown promising results in preliminary studies, and may be of benefit in mild to moderate SLE.

- Corticosteroids are needed infrequently, and should be avoided for the treatment of pain not associated with inflammation. With patients who respond to steroids, we start the patient on an NSAID and hydroxychloroquine and reduce the steroid dose.

- For resistant inflammatory arthritis, methotrexate 7.5 mg/week has been useful in small studies. In one prospective study of 12 patients on high doses of corticosteroids to control primarily arthritic symptoms, 3 patients discontinued methotrexate because of side effects. In six of the remaining nine patients, the corticosteroid dose was reduced by an average of 42 percent.

- Low-dose tricyclic antidepressants (e.g., amitriptyline 5 to 30 mg HS) are often useful when pain has been unresponsive to the above measures.

TREATMENT OF PSYCHIATRIC AND NEUROLOGIC MANIFESTATIONS

Psychosis due to active organic involvement by SLE usually responds to steroids. Treatment should be initiated as soon as possible to prevent permanent damage. Prednisone (1 to 2 mg/kg per day) given for a few weeks in divided doses is usually sufficient. If we see no improvement within two to three weeks, a trial of cytotoxic therapy (e.g., pulse cyclophosphamide) is warranted. One study, for example, evaluated this therapy in thirty-one patients with severe neuropsychiatric lupus who had primarily failed previous therapy with corticosteroids and, in some cases, oral cytotoxic drugs. All patients were treated with intravenous pulse cyclophosphamide; eight patients were treated with plasmapheresis. Substantial improvement was seen in 61 percent and partial improvement in 29 percent.

While waiting for steroids or immunosuppressive drugs to take effect, psychologic manifestations are best treated with antipsychotic drugs (such as haloperidol), as well as with active support by health caretakers and family.

Treatment of cognitive problems is based upon their presumed cause. If due to medications, such as steroids, we consider reducing the dose or stopping therapy. If associated with antiphospholipid antibodies, we begin anticoagulation. If associated with antineuronal antibodies, a short course of steroids (0.5 mg/kg for a few weeks) may be beneficial. Cognitive retraining may be effective in patients with persistent symptoms.

Generalized seizures are usually managed with phenytoin and barbiturates. Partial complex seizures and psychosis related to seizures are best treated with carbamazepine, Klonopin (clonaxepam), valproic acid, and gabapentine. If new onset seizures are thought to reflect an acute inflammatory event, or if a concomitant flare exists, a short course of steroids (prednisone, 1 mg/kg in divided doses) may be given in an attempt to prevent the development of a permanent epileptic focus.

The treatment of headaches in patients with SLE does not differ from that in patients without this disease unless there are other manifestations of CNS lupus as noted above. Most patients respond to NSAIDs and/or acetaminophen. Corticosteroids and narcotics are rarely warranted, although they may be beneficial in patients with severe migraine. Low-dose tricyclic antidepressants (e.g., amitriptyline at 5 to 30 mg per day) are often helpful for frequently occurring headaches.

The role of cyclophosphamide and/or plasmapheresis in the management of CNS lupus is not well defined. We consider these modalities in patients with the following characteristics:

- Acute or recent onset of neurological symptoms, such as seizures or organic brain syndromes, in the absence of another cause.

- Evidence of active inflammation in the brain such as increased cells and protein in the cerebrospinal fluid, brain swelling on MRI or CT scan, vascular injury on MR angiography, and high titer antibrain antibodies.

- Failure to respond to a one- to two-week course of high dose oral corticosteroids (e.g., prednisone in a dose of 1 to 2 mg/kg per day) or to pulse methylprednisolone (1,000 mg/day for three days).

TREATMENT OF CARDIOVASCULAR MANIFESTATIONS

Symptomatic pericarditis often responds to a nonsteroidal anti-inflammatory drug, especially indomethacin. Patients who do not tolerate or respond to a NSAID can be treated with prednisone (0.5 to 1 mg/kg per day in divided doses).

Myocarditis should be treated with prednisone (1 mg/kg per day in divided doses) plus usual therapy for congestive heart failure, if present. A few patients have been treated with cyclophosphamide or azathioprine. Cardiomyopathy is usually resistant to steroids and/or immunosuppressive drugs.

Patients with SLE should be made aware of the importance of risk factor reduction for atherosclerosis/coronary artery disease/"hardening of the arteries." In one study, for example, only 17 percent of the patients believed that they were at high risk for developing coronary artery disease within five years, when, in fact, three or more risk factors were present in 53 percent of patients.

Patients with lupus should be advised to stop smoking, to exercise, and to follow measures designed to improve lipid profiles. Hydroxychloroquine should be used in preference to prednisone whenever possible, and aspirin should be prescribed for its antiplatelet properties.

Hypertension is an important risk factor in SLE. We favor aggressive therapy, aiming for a diastolic pressure below 85 mmHg, especially in younger patients. The choice of antihypertensive agent depends, in part, upon coexisting disorders. We use nifedipine in patients with Raynaud's phenomenon and an angiotensin converting enzyme (ACE) inhibitor in patients with renal disease. Steroids may contribute to hypertension, so the steroid dosage should be reduced, if possible. Symptomatic coronary disease should be treated as it is in patients without lupus.

In postmenopausal women, hormone replacement therapy (HRT) with estrogen and progestin can decrease the risk of both coronary disease and osteoporosis, improve the mood and sense of well-being and libido. However, these benefits must be weighed against the potential risk of exacerbating SLE. Via uncertain mechanisms, estrogen increases the susceptibility to SLE, which probably explains the marked female preponderance in this disorder. However, the risk of HRT appears to be small. One report, for example, compared thirty women on HRT to thirty "never-users." There was no difference in lupus activity between the two groups.

It has also been suggested that hormone replacement therapy may be associated with an increased likelihood of developing SLE. Data from the Nurses' Health Study found that when compared with women who were never treated with estrogen replacement therapy, the relative risk of SLE was 2.5 in current users of HRT and 1.8 in past users.

Similar concerns about exacerbation of SLE have been raised with the use of oral contraceptives. In the past, the use of estrogen-containing oral contraceptives was associated with an increased risk of activation of lupus. However, most currently available oral contraceptives are primarily progesterones and/or low-dose estrogens. These preparations are not generally associated with adverse effects in women with systemic lupus erythematosus. In one report, for example, four of thirty-one women (13 percent) had an exacerbation of lupus within six months after starting an oral contraceptive. Two women treated with an oral contraceptive developed deep venous thrombosis (clotting); both of these women had antiphospholipid antibodies.

Thus, modern oral contraceptives are probably safe in most patients with SLE but should probably be avoided in women already at increased risk of clotting. This includes patients with antiphospholipid antibodies, nephrotic syndrome, and/or a history of thrombophlebitis. Patients with active nephritis also may be at increased risk of renal exacerbation. In these patients, barrier methods, such as condoms, are the contraceptive method of choice, since intrauterine devices can be complicated by hemorrhage or infection.

Chronic warfarin therapy is indicated in most patients with stroke syndromes due to antiphospholipid antibodies or thrombosis once they are stable, and if there is no evidence of hemorrhage. The INR is generally maintained between 3 and 4. The administration of corticosteroids and perhaps cyclophosphamide may be warranted if there is an associated lupus flare (including vasculitis). By contrast, steroids are not used in patients with a stroke and antiphospholipid antibodies but no evidence of active lupus. Steroid therapy is usually ineffective in this setting and may be associated with significant side effects.

TREATING LUPUS SYMPTOMS IN PREGNANT PATIENTS

There are two issues related to therapy of women with lupus who become pregnant: monitoring of disease activity in both asymptomatic and symptomatic patients; and treatment of active disease.

Monitoring

Mothers should be assessed for disease activity at least once each trimester, and more if active. The schedule for monitoring includes:

- Physical examination, including blood pressure
- Renal function—urinalysis, plasma creatinine concentration, and 24-hour urine collection for protein
- Complete blood count, anti-DNA titer, and complement levels
- Pelvic ultrasonography to monitor fetal growth

- Anti-Ro/SSA, anti-La/SSB, and antiphospholipid antibodies (at onset of pregnancy)

Women who show evidence of increased serologic activity but remain asymptomatic should be monitored more closely. We do not initiate therapy for serologic findings alone.

Active Lupus

Treatment of SLE during pregnancy is associated with some unique problems. Consideration must be given to the following issues:

- Medications used to treat SLE may cross the placenta and cause fetal harm. Thus, the risks and benefits of treatment during pregnancy must be repeatedly weighed against the risk of activity of SLE having a deleterious effect on the mother and the fetus.
- Nephritis in pregnancy requires special consideration because of its potential morbidity, and possible confusion with pre-eclampsia.
- Treatment of the other with antiphospholipid antibodies is important because of the risk of both fetal demise and low birth weight.

Medication Use

Medications that are typically used to treat patients with SLE may be divided into three categories: those that should be avoided in pregnancy; those that are probably safe to use in pregnant patients; and those that are safe.

- Medications that may cause birth defects should be avoided, such as cyclophosphamide and methotrexate.
- Antimalarials theoretically may cause problems to the fetus, although none have been documented. Thus, hydrochloroquine is probably safe to use.
- NSAIDs are safe, but should be discontinued in the last few weeks of pregnancy (to facilitate closure of the *ductus arteriosus*—the channel between the mother's pulmonary artery and the fetus's aorta).
- Prednisone is "safe" in that no fetal defects develop other than rare temporary neonatal adrenal suppression. Steroid side effects in the mother may be reduced by recommending a low-salt diet (to prevent weight increase and hypertension), an exercise program (to prevent bone loss and depression), and calcium supplementation (to prevent osteoporosis).
- Azathioprine may be used cautiously.

Serological markers (complement, anti-DNA antibodies) should be monitored closely. Increasing abnormality of these markers is not necessarily a rationale for a change in therapy, but is an indication that closer observation is necessary for possible exacerbation of lupus. If treatment of a flare is deemed necessary, high-dose prednisone is the therapy of choice.

Renal Disease

Patients with a significant flare of lupus nephritis should be treated with high-dose prednisone, antihypertensive medication (e.g., hydralazine, methyldopa, and calcium channel blockers; but not diuretics, ACE inhibitors, or some beta blockers). In addition, the fetus should be delivered as soon as possible. Signs of a renal flare include renewed activity in the urine sediment and an increase in the plasma creatinine concentration. In comparison, an isolated elevation in protein excretion is a common, probably hemodynamically mediated finding in all glomerulopathies during pregnancy and should not necessarily be considered a finding of increased lupus activity.

There is little if any experience with pulse methylprednisolone in pregnancy and its effects on the fetus are unknown. Cyclophosphamide should be avoided if possible during pregnancy, but azathioprine can be used with relative safety as long as the white blood cell count is normal.

Thrombocytopenia

Thrombocytopenia occurring during lupus pregnancies may have multiple causes, including antiplatelet antibodies, toxemia, and antiphospholipid antibodies. Treatment for this disorder includes high-dose prednisone and intravenous immune globulin.

Antiphospholipid Antibody Syndrome

As previously mentioned, patients with antiphospholipid antibodies may be at high risk for recurrent fetal loss, especially during the middle trimester. A detailed discussion of treatment in these patients is discussed elsewhere. The following general recommendations can be made:

- Patients with antiphospholipid antibodies should be managed with subcutaneous heparin (10,000 to 12,000 units twice a day, especially for weeks twelve through thirty-two) plus low-dose aspirin (81 mg/day). Frequent complication of this regimen is heparin-induced osteoporosis. Recovery of bone density occurs postpartum after the heparin is discontinued; it is unclear, however, if the recovery is complete.

- If heparin and aspirin therapy do not prevent fetal loss, intravenous gamma globulin should be tried during the next pregnancy (0.4 g/kg per day for five consecutive days of each month).

- If IVIG (intravenous immune globulin) fails, prednisone (20 to 40 mg/day) and low-dose aspirin can be tried in the next pregnancy, although it may be associated with a high morbidity (the rate of incidence of disease).

Patients with the antiphospholipid syndrome should be monitored carefully by sonography early in pregnancy, and at about twenty weeks for fetal heart rate. Women with a history of intravascular clotting events should probably be anticoagulated for a few months postpartum.

TREATMENT OF CHEST PAIN

Chest wall pain generally responds to local heat, nonsteroidal anti-inflammatory drugs, topical analgesics, and acetaminophen. Local trigger point injections may be helpful in refractory cases; steroids are rarely necessary.

Pleural disease in SLE often responds to therapy with NSAIDs. If there is no response within a few days, moderate to high dose steroids will generally be effective. Immunosuppressive agents are rarely indicated.

TREATMENT OF KIDNEY DISEASE

Optimal therapy of membranous lupus is uncertain. Asymptomatic patients are often not treated, those with moderate disease may be treated with prednisone, while those with a rising plasma creatinine concentration or marked nephrotic syndrome are often treated with the same regimen as diffuse proliferative glomerulonephritis. An NIH (National Institutes of Health) study randomized twenty-two patients with membranous nephropathy but no proliferative disease to one year of prednisone alone, pulse cyclophosphamide (as described below), or cyclosporine (5 mg/kg per day). Each therapy appeared to be effective with cyclophosphamide perhaps being most beneficial.

Protein excretion fell below 2 g/day in fourteen patients: four of eight with prednisone, five of six with cyclophosphamide, and four of five with cyclosporine. All four cyclosporine-treated patients relapsed when therapy was discontinued versus only two of ten receiving other therapies. At one year, six patients (two in each group) had more than a 20-percent rise in glomerular filtration rate, while three (two prednisone, one cyclosporine) had more than a 20-percent fall in glomerular filtration rate. Thus, there was a trend favoring intravenous cyclophosphamide, but more patients must be evaluated to fully define the optimal therapy of this condition.

Although some patients with diffuse proliferative lupus respond to corticosteroids alone, most studies suggest that renal survival is significantly enhanced by the addition of a cytotoxic agent, such as cyclophosphamide. A meta-analysis combining the results of multiple controlled trials found that the addition of cyclophosphamide or azathioprine lowered the incidence of progression to end-stage renal disease by 40 percent when compared with therapy with corticosteroids alone. High-risk patients may derive even greater benefit; in studies performed at the National Institutes of Health, for example, the probability of avoiding renal failure at ten to twelve years in high-risk patients was 90 percent with cyclophosphamide, 60 percent with azathioprine (this was not significantly different from cyclophosphamide), and only 20 percent with prednisone. Although patients may do better with azathioprine than prednisone alone during the first ten years of follow-up, there is no longer significant difference in the incidence of renal failure in the longer term and the results are clearly *inferior* to those in patients initially treated with cyclophosphamide.

These trials also suggest that, rather than being given orally on a daily basis (2 to 2.5 mg/kg per day), cyclophosphamide may be less toxic when given as monthly intravenous boluses (doses injected all at once): beginning with 0.75 g/m$_2$ of body surface area and, assuming the white blood cell count remains above 3,000/mm$_3$, increasing to a maximum of 1 g/m$_2$ given in a saline solution over thirty to sixty minutes. Even obese patients have generally been treated according to body surface area; a lower initial dose of 0.5 g/m$_2$ minimizes the risk of overdosing in this setting. An oral pulse cyclophosphamide regimen may also be effective but this regimen is still experimental.

Plasmapheresis

Plasmapheresis appears to be of no added benefit to immunosuppressive therapy in most patients. A randomized controlled trial of 86 patients with severe lupus nephritis showed that treatment with plasmapheresis, prednisone, and short-term oral cyclophosphamide led to a more rapid decline in circulating autoantibody levels (such as anti-double-stranded DNA antibodies) but no difference in outcome when compared with treatment with prednisone and cyclophosphamide alone. The percentage of patients progressing to renal failure (25 percent versus 17 percent) and going into clinical remission (30 percent versus 28 percent) was virtually the same in both groups.

These findings do not mean that selected patients might not benefit from plasmapheresis. It has also been suggested that the regimen used was not optimized to prevent rebound autoantibody production, thereby minimizing its possible efficacy. One study of fourteen patients with severe lupus (and active but not severe lupus nephritis) refractory to conventional immunosuppressive therapy utilized the following aggressive regimen. Although this preliminary uncontrolled observation cannot be routinely recommended, all fourteen patients responded and eight remained *off therapy* for five to six years.

- Cytotoxic agents gradually withdrawn to ensure maximum lymphocyte activation, and corticosteroids were stopped two days prior to therapy.

- Plasmapheresis, in which 60 ml/kg was removed and replaced with albumin, was performed on days one through three.

- Pulse intravenous cyclophosphamide, 12 ml/kg, was given six hours after the last plasmapheresis on day three and then on days four and five.

- Oral cyclophosphamide was begun on day six at a dose of 1 mg/kg per day, and after the white cell count had increased to above 2,000, 2 to 5 mg/kg per day for two to five months to maintain the white cell count between 2,000 and 5,000.

- Oral prednisone was begun at a dose of 2 mg/kg per day on days five through seven, 1 mg/kg per day on day eight and then gradually tapered at a rate of approximately 0.1 mg/kg per day per week.

The main side effects were five episodes of herpes zoster and four women developed irreversible amenorrhea. One patient had a major relapse, and two others had minor relapses at two and three years.

Intravenous Immune Globulin

The administration of intravenous immune globulin (IVIG) can diminish immunologic activity in certain autoimmune diseases, perhaps by interacting with Fc receptors on effector cells or by the presence of anti-idiotypic antibodies directed against idiotypes on the patient's own autoantibodies. A small uncontrolled study of nine resistant patients found that IVIG led to histologic, immunologic, and clinical improvement. However, other observations in lupus nephritis suggest that disease activity may be increased, perhaps due to enhanced immune complex formation mediated by the infused IgG (immunoglobulin G). Thus, the efficacy of this regimen must be evaluated in controlled studies.

Cyclosporine

There is only a limited reported experience with cyclosporine in lupus nephritis. One uncontrolled trial, for example, consisted of the administration of cyclosporine and steroids in patients resistant to cytotoxic therapy. This regimen led to reductions in clinical activity, proteinuria, and histologic activity without any worsening of the plasma creatinine concentration at two year follow-up.

A second study treated ten patients with nephrotic syndrome and membranous nephropathy with cyclosporine, usually in combination with low-dose prednisone, for three to four years. All patients had decreased lupus activity and a substantial reduction in proteinuria; six went into complete remission. Three patients had a lupus flare during therapy that responded to standard treatment, such as increasing the dose of prednisone. Repeat renal biopsy in five patients showed decreased active disease but more advanced interstitial fibrosis, presumably due to scarring of the previous inflammatory injury.

Future controlled studies should elucidate the efficacy of cyclosporine in lupus nephritis. At present, it is a reasonable consideration in patients with refractory disease or those who cannot tolerate more conventional therapies. Cost is always an important issue with cyclosporine. Studies in adult renal transplant recipients suggest that the concurrent administration of the antifungal agent ketoconazole markedly diminishes the cyclosporine dose by slowing hepatic metabolism and reduces the total cost (cyclosporine plus ketoconazole versus cyclosporine alone) by over 70 percent. A similar but less pronounced effect can be attained with the calcium channel blockers diltiazem and verapamil.

Total Lymphoid Irradiation

Total lymphoid irradiation (as used in Hodgkin's disease) may induce remission of clinical and serologic disease. This aggressive regimen, however, has not been widely evaluated.

TREATMENT OF EPIDERMAL LESIONS

The goal of treatment in the different forms of cutaneous lupus is to prevent long-term skin sequelae (secondary conditions), such as telangiectasia (dilation of a group of capillaries), hyperpigmentation or hypopigmentation, alopecia, and scarring.

Prevention

Preventive measures will prevent skin lesions in most patients. Those who are photosensitive should be taught to avoid high sun exposure (beaches, snow, lakes), especially between 10 A.M. and 3 P.M., and, if possible, medications that may cause photosensitivity.

Photosensitive patients should also use sunscreens daily. The sunscreen should be applied thirty to sixty minutes prior to exposure and reapplied every four to six hours. Sunscreens of at least SPF 15 should be used; higher SPFs are available for more sensitive patients.

Treatment

Mucous membrane lesions respond well to topical steroids and systemic antimalarial drugs. The response to topical steroids (usually Orabase with either hydrocortisone or triamcinolone) takes a few days to weeks, while the response to hydroxychloroquine takes weeks to months.

Telangiectasia requires no specific therapy, other than make-up for the concerned individual. A green foundation (to neutralize the red) followed by the makeup color of choice usually suffices. Current cutaneous lasers, such as the tunable dye, are very effective in removing telangiectasias.

Raynaud's phenomenon often be prevented by educating the patient about preventing trigger factors such as avoidance of smoking, caffeine, vasopressors, vasoconstrictors, and for cold-induced Raynaud's, wearing warm clothing (such as thermal underwear, mittens, and hats). More severe or resistant disease can be treated with vasodilators, such as nifedipine or nicardipine, topical nitroglycerine, and/or prazosin. Intravascular treatment with prostacyclin may be required in some cases.

Topical Therapy

A lupus rash should initially be treated with topical corticosteroids. *Hydrocortisone* will often suffice, but more potent steroids (particularly the fluorinated preparations) are available for thicker lesions. There are several points that deserve emphasis:

- Fluorinated steroids may be used for facial lesions, but should be used very cautiously and probably for no more than two weeks.
- Ointments are more effective than creams.
- Lotions should be used on scalp lesions.
- Chronic use of topical steroids may lead to skin atrophy, thinning, telangiectasia, hypertrichosis (excessive hair growth for certain areas of the body), striae (the appearance of bands or stripes on the skin), and depigmentation.

Antimalarial Drugs

Patients with persistent rashes should be treated with an antimalarial. These drugs should be used only when the diagnosis is secure with the following precautions:

- They have been associated with flares of psoriasis.
- Antimalarial drugs should not be given to the rare individual with G6PD deficiency.
- They may cause serious eye changes, including macular degeneration; as a result, all patients should have retinal examinations at six month intervals.

Currently, the most popular antimalarial in SLE is hydroxychloroquine (200 to 400 mg/day). In one study, for example, overall improvement of erythema, infiltration, scaling, and hyperkeratosis occurred in 50 percent of patients. Chloroquine (250 to 500 mg/day) is somewhat more potent but has a higher risk of eye damage. It produces an anti-inflammatory effect by binding to dermal keratinocytes and thereby presumably decreasing cellular infiltration after UV exposure. Quinacrine (100 mg/day) is even more effective and has a much lower risk of eye damage; however, the skin turns somewhat yellow in most patients and bone marrow depression is a rare complication. Improvement with antimalarials may not be seen until six to twelve weeks of use.

SCLE (subcutaneous lupus) and lupus panniculitis (inflammation of the subcutaneous layer of connective tissue and fat of the abdominal wall) respond best to antimalarial drugs, but higher doses may be needed. Combination therapy with chloroquine and quinacrine was found to be effective among most patients with chronic cutaneous lupus and/or SCLE resistant to antimalarial monotherapy.

Systemic Agents

Systemic steroids and immunosuppressive agents are rarely needed to clear skin lesions except for bullous lesions (those with blisters). Some dermatologists favor local injections of resistant lesions with corticosteroids. Systemic drugs that have been used when local therapy fails include oral steroids, dapsone, azathioprine, thalidomide, gold, retinoids, methotrexate, cyclophosphamide, chlorambucil, intravenous immune globulin, diphenylhydantoin, anti-CD4 antibodies, and clofazimine.

Cosmetic Treatment of Skin Manifestations

Erythematous lesions can be disguised with the use of cosmetics such as Cover Mark, Dermablend, or a green foundation.

TREATMENT OF GASTROINTESTINAL MANIFESTATIONS

Treatment of esophageal symptoms depends upon the specific etiology. Dysmotility is treated with cisapride (10 mg four times per day) as with other causes of dysmotility. Esophageal stricture is treated by endoscopic dilatation and/or eating frequent small meals. Symptoms due to GERD (gastroesophageal reflux disease) may be treated with reflux precautions (e.g., elevating the head of the bed, avoiding lying down after meals), and the administration of antacids, H2 antagonists, or a proton pump inhibitor (e.g., omeprazole). Esophageal candidiasis is treated with nystatin or fluconazole.

The dyspepsia attributed to corticosteroids or NSAIDs may respond to medical withdrawal. If NSAIDs must be continued or symptoms persist, the patient can be treated with one or more of the following:

- Antacids.
- H2 blockers, which can be associated with healing of ulcers even when NSAID therapy is continued.
- *Helicobacter pylori* infection should be looked for and treated in patients with peptic ulcers (particularly duodenal ulcers).
- Cessation of cigarette smoking and excess alcohol consumption should always be recommended.

Prophylactic therapy also may be beneficial in certain settings. As an example, I generally recommend either misoprostol (200 micrograms three to four times per day with meals) or H2 blockers in patients requiring NSAIDs who have a history of dyspepsia. Many doctors also routinely treat patients treated with high dose steroids (60 mg of prednisone per day or its equivalent) with an H2 blocker to "prevent" peptic disease. H2 blockers are recommended because the anti-inflammatory effect of the steroids can easily mask a perforation.

32

Psychiatric Side Effects of Medicines Used in S.L.E.

by Howard S. Shapiro, M.D.

The many different medications used in SLE often produce side effects that alter the patient's thinking, mood, emotional control, and behavior. Any of these effects may be difficult to distinguish from a concurrent anxious or depressed condition or from the lupus itself.

Because of the broad variation of organ system involvement from case to case in SLE, as well as variations in medication programs, underlying personalities, and psychosocial stresses associated with the chronic illness state, determining the cause of psychiatric side effects (PSE) in SLE may be quite challenging. Complicating this is the fact that medications frequently interact with one another.

Liver or kidney involvement may have a profound effect upon the psyche, since these organs are involved in the metabolism and filtering of medications from the blood.

Some drugs *decrease* other drugs' potency and effect, whereas others may *increase* other drugs' potency and effect. Of course, many medications do not interact with one another. Often, a medication that has some predictable side effect is used for a brief period of time, since its undesirable side effect is significantly outweighed by its desired benefit. Given this complicated picture, you can see that it helps to understand the various possible psychological effects of your medications, as well as potential drug interactions.

SALICYLATES

Salicylates, such as aspirin, may have been used longer than any other drugs to reduce inflammation. The side effects of high doses (up to 3 to 6 grains per day) are well known, such as gastrointestinal injury with hidden and unrecognized bleeding, reduced blood clotting (thinning of the blood), and disturbances in liver function. Less well known is that chronic use of salicylates can lead to toxic blood levels associated with ringing in the ears (tinnitus), confusion, and visual and auditory hallucinations, which can be confused with a psychosis or even lupus cerebritis. Hyperventilation may occur, leading to lightheadedness, vertigo, dizziness, headaches, fainting, and possible accidents. This is especially true in older patients in whom it may easily be misinterpreted as Alzheimer's disease.

NSAIDS

Nowadays, drugs such as indomethacin and phenylbutazone are rarely used. However, there are newer nonsteroidal anti-inflammatory drugs (NSAIDs)—including piroxicam, sulindac, ibuprofen, naproxen, meclofenamate, tolmetin, and fenoprofen—that can be tried at some point during the illness. Their side effects are similar and usually less than that seen with aspirin. They may have effects upon kidney filtration and function and some have potential for CNS side effects. There are many reports in the medical literature of CNS dysfunction in all age groups due to NSAIDs. Tolmetin has been reported as inducing mania in a patient with a prior history of recurrent major depression and hypomanic episodes. Like other NSAIDs, tolmetin is associated with a variety of neurosensory side effects, such as headache, drowsiness, blurred vision, and dizziness. Tinnitus occurs in as many as 13 percent of cases.

Depression also has been associated with some of the NSAIDs, especially with ibuprofen, fenoprofen, and naproxen. Ibuprofen, now available without a prescription and packaged under different trade names, has been linked to a few psychotic reactions, as has sulindac (closely related to indomethacin). While the exact mechanism for the CNS action in NSAIDs is not certain, they are known to cross the blood-brain barrier and, in part, have an analgesic and anti-fever action upon the hypothalamus. They work by inhibiting prostaglandin production in the brain, which modulates the effect of various neurotransmitters.

ANTIMALARIALS

The antimalarial drugs, especially chloroquine, have been associated with a number of psychiatric reactions when taken in high doses. Generally speaking, the "mild side effects," such as tiredness and depression occur more frequently with chloroquine (40 percent) than with hydroxychloroquine (29 percent). One study found that 50 percent to 60 percent of sixty-five patients with rheumatic diseases experienced side effects from antimalarial drugs, such as severe depression, confusional states, depersonalization, psychosis with hallucinations, and sleep difficulty. The latter may be related to visual field and/or optic nerve changes.

CYTOTOXIC DRUGS

Chemotherapy with immunosuppressive agents, such as those used in cancer, are administered occasionally to lupus patients resistant to other forms of therapy. These drugs, called cytotoxic and/or antineoplastic agents, include methotrexate, azathioprine, and cyclophosphamide. Their toxic effects target young, rapidly growing cells, such as those in the bloodstream and immune, gastrointestinal, and reproductive systems. The physical side effects are more serious than the psychological side effects and include hepatitis, increased risk of infection, and hemorrhagic cystitis (especially with cyclophosphamide).

At lower oral doses, no direct psychiatric side effects have been noted from immunosuppressives with the exception of methotrexate, where headache was a common side effect.

STEROIDS

Oral steroids (prednisone, prednisolone) are frontline treatment for SLE. Steroids have been used in many conditions and their effects studied extensively. Intra-articular injections are common in acutely inflamed, uninfected joints. Long-term oral use is known to produce psychiatric side effects as well as a series of organic side effects, such as increased risk of infection, muscle deterioration, cataracts, increased appetite and weight gain, osteoporosis, aseptic necrosis, and redistribution of fat with changes in figure and form, as well as hormonal and metabolic changes, just to mention a few.

Short-term use may be necessary for flares of unremitting pericarditis, pleuritis, scleritis, vasculitis, encephalitis, prolonged fever, and/or serious blood changes. The medical literature is filled with studies indicating that approximately 5 to 10 percent of patients treated with steroids, including ACTH (adrenocortitropic hormone, or cortisone), developed severe psychiatric syndromes. By and large, the medical literature states that the most common side effect of steroids is depression. Hyperactivity, tension, and hypomania occur less frequently, and psychotic reactions are less likely; delirium and disorientation are even less common. In general, steroid reactions occur soon after the drugs are started, primarily within the first few weeks.

Symptoms like these are usually, but not always, reversible when the medication is withdrawn. Manic and hypomanic reactions have been more apt to be noticed than depressive reactions, since they reflect a more marked alteration in customary personality, whereas depressive reactions are often less noticeable and easy to conceal. It is as if one expects depression in a "sick" person. The higher the prednisone dosage, the greater the likelihood of psychiatric symptoms, although there are a few cases of profound personality changes due to small doses.

DRUGS USED TO TREAT PSYCHIATRIC MANIFESTATIONS

Because of the frequent occurrence, incipient nature, and camouflaged presentation of CNS involvement in lupus, there is often uncertainty as to whether a "psychiatric" reaction is drug-induced, due to the lupus itself, due to the stress and strains and sacrifices of being ill, or due to something that would have happened, even if there had been no lupus. (If you think you're confused at this point, imagine how the doctor feels . . . especially when caring for a new patient.) The physician who knows his/her patient's persona and customary mental status has a big edge in recognizing, evaluating, and treating the lupus patient who has had a relatively sudden alteration in psyche.

Because depression, anxiety manifestations, sleep disturbances, hypersensitivity, diminished emotional control, and other neurological side effects occur not infrequently in the lives of lupus patients, it is not surprising that physicians prescribe a number of specific psychopharmacological agents, such as minor tranquilizers, hypnotics, antianxiety agents, sedatives, various types of antidepressants, analgesics (painkillers), muscle relaxants, beta-blockers, and psychostimulants, to mention just a few.

Benzodiazepines

The most frequently prescribed medication for anxiety and tension is in the class called benzodiazepines. There are many different brands, which vary from one another in their speed of onset of action, duration of action, ways they interact with other drugs, and potential for dependency and habituation (addiction). They are used temporarily for acute anxiety associated with specific procedures, such as joint fluid needling. They may be used in sleep disturbances, which is a common experience in SLE patients, and often they are used for the anxiety that frequently develops secondarily to an unremitting depression. Anxiety often develops when there is a chronic source of discomfort, such as musculoskeletal pain, fatigue state, and/or chronic impairment of sleep and rest patterns. The principal indication for their use is reduction of unbearable anxiety, especially when anxiety is making the patient dysfunctional.

Media attention has focused on the rapid-acting benzodiazepines, especially alprazolam (Xanax) and triazolam (Halcion) and the possible undesirable effects that these medications have on rare occasions. Occasionally, these medications disrupt memory and other cognitive functions, most notably attention, concentration, reasoning, and short-term memory and recall to a significant degree. This is especially significant because, in a lupus patient, these changes could easily be mistaken for subclinical CNS involvement. Perhaps more significant, these medications may intensify any pre-existing symptoms of impaired cognition due to lupus itself.

Benzodiazepines can be given safely to SLE patients, provided kidney and liver function are intact. Other medications that may alter the effect of benzodiazepines are cimetidine and immunosuppressive drugs, such as methotrexate. These can impair liver function, thereby slowing the breakdown of other drugs and increasing the duration and strength of their effect. Patients with vasculitis or renal damage may have difficulty in excreting the breakdown products in the urine. Side effects, such as sedation, depression, and disturbances in balance, movement, and gait, should be accounted for with careful adjustment in dosage.

Barbiturates

The barbiturates have little place in medical management these days because of their high potential for abuse and their lethality when taken in overdose or in conjunction with alcohol and/or other CNS depressants. Moreover, they stimulate the liver to more rapidly metabolize a number of other medications taken by the SLE patient, such as corticosteroids, and thereby decrease their effect.

Antidepressants

Many studies indicate that major depressive disorders in the medically ill are undertreated and inadequately treated even when recognized. It is not uncommon to misdiagnose a depressive reaction as a lupus flare-up, since many features are similar, such as fatigue, insomnia, anorexia, anxiety, pain intensification, and social withdrawal. Depressive reactions, in and of themselves, are very stressful and anxiety-producing, and may exacerbate lupus. So as not to confuse cause with effect, a careful physical examination and history along with serial laboratory monitoring is essential. The physician must treat a depressive reaction with the same aggressiveness and persistence as he or she would treat, for example, congestive heart failure or increased intracranial pressure that was not responding to conventional treatment.

Antidepressant medication is the major class of drugs used to treat major depressive reactions. Antidepressants can be divided into four categories: tricyclics, newer generation and non-tricyclic antidepressants, MAO inhibitors, and lithium. There are many different brands of antidepressants today, all of which have one thing in common: all are associated with marked side effects of varying types. When they are effective, there is a dramatic and welcomed improvement in the patient's well-being, and in their symptoms. One antidepressant or combination of antidepressants may work where another has been ineffective or given in an insufficient dose. One of the major side effects (the anti-cholinergic effect) of the antidepressants is that they exacerbate dryness of the mouth, eyes, and vagina that can be associated with SLE. Since many patients are already using saliva-stimulating lozenges and artificial tear treatment, they can tolerate the effect of the antidepressants. While alprazolam is the only option without the anticholinergic side effect, it lacks a strong antidepressant effect in most patients. Nortriptyline, imipramine, and desipramine, in sufficient doses have been well tolerated, although they tend to be sedating, as are ixopepin, amitriptyline, and trazodone. Trazodone has been associated with prominent orthostatic hypotension, which may lead to fainting. Antidepressants do not ordinarily have serious interaction problems with the drugs used in SLE, as long as liver and kidney function are not impaired. Side effects may be intolerable to some patients and require shifting to a different medication.

Lithium carbonate is used to prevent and treat mood disorders, such as recurrent manic illness (bipolar and unipolar), as well as acute mania. The aforementioned may occur in patients with SLE because lithium is excreted through the kidneys and itself has a profound effect upon kidney function. Its use, in lupus patients, must be as a last choice, with great caution, and for brief periods of time. When lithium is used, frequent careful urine, blood, and renal function tests are necessary, as well as careful neuropsychiatric evaluation. The excretion of lithium could be a problem in a person using NSAIDs, since lithium itself can cause kidney damage, such as interstitial fibrosis or glomerular sclerosis, and thereby confound the monitoring of kidney function. Nephrogenic diabetes insipidus induced by lithium might cause the elimination of other medications. Lithium can induce hypothyroidism, which could easily be missed in a patient on maintenance steroid-therapy and/or in a depressed individual. Finally, lithium concentrations in the blood may be raised to toxic levels by drug interactions with ibuprofen, piroxicam, indomethacin, and others; they act by decreasing elimination of lithium in the kidney, thereby increasing the concentration of lithium in the serum.

To my mind, lithium is indicated as an anti-manic prophylaxis in a patient who must be given steroids when the patient has an established history of severe and dangerous manic reaction/response to corticosteroids (such as after pulse therapy) or in a lupus patient with no psychiatric history who develops an unexplained and unmanageable manic reaction that has not responded within forty-eight hours to a significant increase or decrease in steroid dosage or to other antipsychotic medications (neuroleptics).

Narcotics

Generally, when one refers to painkillers, he or she means agents other than nonsteroidal anti-inflammatory drugs (NSAIDs), which have a double analgesic pathway. The other painkillers are mostly derivatives of, or chemical equivalents of, more potent and powerfully acting narcotics; items of this class include codeine, oxycodone and aspirin (Percodan), pentazocine hydrochloride and aspirin (Talwin), and mesperidine hydrochloride (Demerol). There is a high potential for dependency and habituation to these agents, especially since they have antidepressant and anti-anxiety effects. Because of what is called the rapid development of "tolerance" (whereby a greater and greater amount of medication is required to elicit the desired effect), the user finds that any interruption in the continued use of the drug produces withdrawal. Withdrawal is characterized by a rebound exacerbation of the original symptoms for which the drugs were used in the first place, for example, the pain-anxiety-pain cycle. This very unpleasant withdrawal reaction drives an individual to continued use of these narcotic substances; in fact, the user is now taking the substance not for its original purpose, but to feel "okay" by warding off the withdrawal reaction; it becomes a vicious and cruel cycle.

Psychic Energizers

Another class of substances occasionally misused and/or misprescribed in SLE are called psychic energizers. These compounds were popular and prescribed frequently in the past as appetite suppressants and stimulants; there were and still are many different types of chemicals varying from the very potent amphetamines and derivatives to much less potent agents. Their potential for misuse—often quite innocent and even at the suggestion of well-intended caretakers—has become the subject of many movies, books, and TV dramas. Their potential for rapid and profound dependency and habituation is well known. Especially prominent in the histories of users of stimulants is the eventual use of sedatives, hypnotics, and assorted "downers" to neutralize the undesired and uncontrolled duration and degree of action of the stimulants. Since stimulants produce a false sense of energy, enthusiasm, quick or creative thought processes, false sense of well being, and an urge toward action (especially toward physical activity) it is not surprising that the lupus patient finds favor with stimulants. Indeed, many gentle, kind, and caring physicians with good intentions believe that these medications, if and when used occasionally can provide the patient with an occasional "pick-me-up." Furthermore, the physician's permissiveness and good intentions reinforce the patient's innocent acceptance of the use of stimulants as helpful and appropriate and consequence-free. Admittedly for some, this is true. Experience has shown, however, that misuse is the rule, habituation develops rapidly, and the use of stimulants has two other major consequences for the lupus patient. First, the use of stimulants leads to the use of downer drugs and the vicious cycle discussed earlier. Second, and perhaps more serious, stimulant use in the lupus patient frequently leads to exhaustion and burn-out because of overactivity driven by a chemically induced false sense of energy, ambition, and restlessness. This hyper-stimulating state ends in a "crash" and/or burn-out, which may exacerbate a lupus flare, as well as stimulate cravings for more of the stimulants.

Because lupus may be a multi-system condition requiring one of a variety of medications with potential side effects and interactions upon one another, it always behooves the informed patient to learn as much as possible about the medications she or he takes.

33

Placebos

by Robert S. Katz, M.D.

Placebos are inactive substances used as medication. They are not believed by the physician to be effective therapy for a given condition but are used for their psychological effect.

Placebos are often utilized as part of clinical research trials to be compared with a new medication. These research trials demonstrate whether the new medication is truly effective or only equal in value to the placebo. Most research trials use this "blind" approach to test new medications. If neither the physician nor the patient know whether the patient receives an active drug or a placebo, the research trial is known as a "double-blind placebo-controlled study." Such studies are taking place or about to start for several new drugs for lupus patients, including LJP 394, anti-cd40 monoclonal antibodies, and the hormone DHEA. These double-blind studies will accurately assess the true value of these new medications.

Placebos provide a benchmark for measuring the value of medicines. But placebos are actually reasonably effective. If scientists compare individuals receiving a placebo to those taking no medication, the placebo group generally does better. Placebos don't actually help lupus or other diseases, but they can influence the way patients perceive their illness. Like regular exercise or falling in love, placebos influence the way we feel about our condition.

Placebos probably work on brain chemicals, but first one has to have faith in a placebo's possible benefits. "If you don't believe it, it doesn't work," said David Morris in *The Culture of Pain.* Going to a healing professional at a respected medical institution reinforces the effect of any treatment. The expectations of the patient, the impressiveness of a treatment, the expense, the level of concern and attention, and the prestige of the doctor all enhance treatment results. Studies show that when the physician tells a patient that he or she is likely to improve in a few weeks, the benefit is great compared with telling a similar individual that the cause of symptoms is unknown or the course is unpredictable. Placebos are helpful for research purposes but are probably unacceptable as part of standard medical practice because they involve deception, which undermines trust.

Placebos' response rates vary, but can frequently be much higher than the sometimes mentioned figure of one-third. One medical writer Howard Spiro observes that "skeptics have long noted that an operation, particularly a new one, seems to bring benefit for several years until it is reevaluated and then often abandoned."

All of us respond, to one degree or another, to placebos. A placebo responder personality has not been identified, although some studies suggest that those with greater anxiety may be more likely to improve.

Patients with lupus often have fluctuating symptoms and seek medical care or enroll in research studies when their symptoms are at a peak. Because the next step may be for the lupus symptoms to improve spontaneously, this can be misinterpreted as being due to treatment. Placebo-controlled studies sort this out.

Placebos may have dose-response effects: Two placebo tablets may work better than one, or may cause more side effects. Typical side effects in those taking placebos include nausea, fatigue, drowsiness, nervousness, and headaches. For example, headaches were reported by 70 percent of students told that a nonexistent electric current was passed through their heads.

Larger capsules are thought to be stronger. White tablets are often believed to be pain killers. Injections are perceived as "stronger" than pills.

Expectations are important in influencing placebo responses. If individuals are told that a substance is very effective, they respond better than when told the same substance is probably ineffective or might make them worse. A health professional's friendliness and warmth may positively impact a patient's response to both active new drugs and to placebos. Encouragement exerts a placebo effect.

Placebos can sometimes get people to change behavior, and this in turn can lead to a positive treatment response. For example, those with fatigue and achy joints may decide to resume an exercise program, whereas previously they avoided exercise because of pain or fear. Past positive responses to treatment, such as penicillin for strep throat or help from pain killers, may influence patients to associate the relief of symptoms with medications and physician encounters.

Placebos help measure the value of new treatments for lupus. But in their own right they are effective. Whether in the form of tablets, injections, surgery, or positive words and a caring attitude, they can contribute to the effectiveness of treatment. Perhaps they shouldn't be so disparaged and stigmatized. For instance, the therapeutic alliance between doctor and patient produces a placebo effect that helps healing.

34

Laboratory Tests in Lupus

by Michael D. Lockshin, M.D., F.A.C.P.

Are you confused by the names of the blood tests doctors use to diagnose or monitor lupus? Do you know what the tests mean? If you are confused, perhaps the information below will help.

An antibody is a protein (such as gamma globulin and other globulins) that the body normally makes to defend itself against bacteria (germs), viruses, and other things that cause harm. In lupus, the body mistakenly makes antibodies against a person's normal tissue. An antibody is named according to the substance (antigen) against which it is made to fight. Thus, an antibody induced by a polio vaccination is called an anti-polio virus antibody.

Because the basic abnormality of lupus is an immune system that is in overdrive, most of the tests measure the degree to which the immune system is active. Other tests measure the function of specific organs such as the kidneys.

A lot of these tests and names are confusing. Don't worry about such designations as "mg/dL" (milligrams per deciliter). These are technical terms that refer to a specific way of measuring one or another substance. Some laboratories use international units (IUs); some laboratories report the results of chemical tests in molecules (mols) instead of milligrams. I've given the measurements that are most often used. If your laboratory reports your results in a different way, ask your doctor to explain which units are used and what is normal for that laboratory. I have not given numbers for tests that are either reported as positive or negative, or in cases where there are too many ways of reporting to summarize briefly.

Keep in mind that the statements above are just rough guides. There are always exceptions to every rule. I've listed the most common tests and the most common uses, but they may differ for you. If you are still confused, or if you are in doubt, ask your doctor for an explanation.

ANA, FANA

This test looks for antinuclear antibodies, or antibodies against the nucleus, or central controlling part of each cell. (It is also called the fluorescent antinuclear antibody test—FANA.) All organs are made of cells, and all cells have nuclei (plural for nucleus). ANAs have four basic patterns that describe the way they look under a microscope. The patterns are "diffuse" (the whole nucleus lights up), "peripheral" or "rim" (only the ring around the nucleus does), "speckled" (just what it sounds like) and "nucleolar" (two very specific spots light up).

What a Positive Test Means

Almost all patients with lupus have a strongly positive test (still positive even when diluted more than 100 times, commonly expressed 1:100). Many normal people also have positive tests, usually less strong (diluted ten to thirty times, 1:10, 1:30). The diffuse and speckled patterns are common in lupus but are also seen in other diseases and in normals; the peripheral pattern is relatively specific for lupus. The "nucleolar" does not often occur in lupus. A positive test means lupus is a possible diagnosis.

What a Negative Test Means

A negative test usually means that a patient does not have lupus, or that lupus is in remission. However, most patients in remission do not have negative ANAs.

ANTI-(DS)-DNA ANTIBODY

This tests for antibodies to double-stranded (also called native) deoxyribonucleic acid (DNA). DNA is the major part of the cell nucleus, and is the stuff of which our genes are made. The anti-DNA antibody is usually the reason for the positive ANA. People who have a positive ANA who do not have anti-DNA have antibodies against other parts of the nucleus. Anti-ss-DNA (single stranded, or denatured) is less important than anti-ds-DNA.

What a Positive Test Means

An unequivocally positive test in a person with symptoms almost always means lupus is present. The higher the amount, the more likely the disease is active. Rarely, well blood relatives of lupus patients have positive tests, as do some patients with other rare diseases. (There are several ways of expressing a positive test.)

What a Negative Test Means

A negative test does not mean that lupus is not present, since other tests can still be positive in a person who has a positive test, a negative test usually means remission. (See anti-Sm.)

ANTI-SM

This test is designed to look for antibodies to the Smith antigen (named after the patient in whom it was first described). The Smith antigen is a protein that helps DNA stay in its correct shape as it goes about its business directing the cell how to do its work. Together, anti-Sm, anti-RNP, anti-Ro/SSA, and anti La/SSB (see below) are known as "ENA" antigens.

What a Positive Test Means

Like anti-DNA, this test generally means that lupus is present. False positive tests are very rare.

What a Negative Test Means

A negative test does not mean that lupus is not present, since other tests can still be positive. Most persons with lupus have either anti-DNA or anti-Sm antibodies. Negative tests for both generally mean that lupus is not present.

ANTI-RNP

This is a test for antibodies to ribonucleoprotein. The RNP antigen is similar to the Smith antigen, but has a different job in the cell.

What a Positive Test Means

A positive test occurs in some patients with lupus but also in other related diseases. It helps to classify a patient, but it is not usually useful to make a specific diagnosis nor to follow for worsening or recovery.

What a Negative Test Means

A negative test excludes a related disease (mixed connective tissue disease, or MCTD).

ANTI-RO, ANTI-SSA

This test looks for antibodies to the Rose antigen (named after the first patient in whom it was described) and antibodies to the Sjögren's syndrome A antigen. The test was described simultaneously in both lupus and the related disease Sjögren's syndrome (arthritis, dry eyes, dry mouth). The Ro/SSA antigen is similar to the Smith antigen, but has a different job in the cell.

What a Positive Test Means

The test is often positive in lupus patients and in patients with other related diseases. In pregnant women, it may cause a complication known as neonatal lupus. About one-quarter of women with this antibody have a child who develops neonatal lupus.

What a Negative Test Means

If both this test and the related anti-La/SSB test are negative, the child of a pregnant woman will not develop neonatal lupus.

ANTI-LA, ANTI-SSB

These tests look for antibodies to the Lane antigen (named after the first patient in whom it was described) and antibodies to the Sjögren's syndrome B antigen. It is similar to the Ro/SSA antigen.

What a Positive Test Means

The test is often positive in lupus patients and in patients with other related diseases. In pregnant women, it may cause neonatal lupus.

What a Negative Test Means

If both this test and the related anti-Ro/SSA test are negative, the child of a pregnant woman will not develop neonatal lupus.

COMPLEMENT, CH, C3, C4

Complement is a series of proteins that help antibodies fight antigens. CH refers to the amount of complement necessary to destroy (hemolyse) 50 percent of red blood cells in an immune reaction. C3 and C4 are the third and fourth components (of more than 12) of the complement proteins. Complement is used up in immune reactions, such as lupus.

What a Positive Test Means

Low levels of complement mean the body is undergoing a severe immune reaction, primarily in the kidneys. Lupus is one cause, but there are many others. CH is usually 150 to 300 units. C3 about 80 to 150 mg/dL, and C4 about 15 to 40 mg/dL.

What a Negative Test Means

Normal levels of complement make lupus inflammatory kidney disease unlikely. Other types of kidney disease, such as leaky kidneys or scarring, can still occur even if complement is normal. Other types of lupus (rash, arthritis, brain disease) do not usually lower complement.

ACL AND RELATED TESTS

ACL is a test for antibody to cardiolipin. Other related tests include aPL (antibody to phospholipid), the lupus anticoagulant, aPTT (activated partial thromboplastic time), and dRVVT (dilute Russell viper venom time). Cardiolipin is a phospholipid (a type of fat that contains phosphate). There are many other phospholipids, but cardiolipin is the one most frequently tested. The membranes that surround all cells are composed of phospholipids. The test can be performed on clotted blood. The lupus anticoagulant test (for antibodies to clotting factors) can be performed only on fresh blood, since it measures the time it takes the blood to clot. Except for the different techniques, the tests measure approximately, but not exactly, the same things, so it is possible to have a positive aPL test and a negative lupus anticoagulant, and vice versa. APTT and dRVVT are two specific clotting tests used to screen for a lupus anticoagulant antibody.

What a Positive Test Means

An unequivocally and repeatedly positive test means a higher than normal likelihood of developing internal blood clots or problems with pregnancies. Weakly positive tests that come and go are common and generally not important. About one-third of lupus patients have a positive aPL or lupus anticoagulant test. Normal aCL (immunoglobulin G, IgG) is usually under 15 GPL units, for immunoglobulin M (IgM), under 10 MPL units. Normal aPTT is usually under thirty-five seconds.

What a Negative Test Means

A negative test markedly reduces the likelihood of internal clotting problems or certain types of pregnancy complications.

BUN, CREATININE, CREATININE CLEARANCE

Blood urea nitrogen (BUN) and creatinine are chemicals normally excreted by the kidneys. These tests measure the excretion of these chemicals. Creatinine clearance determines how much creatinine the kidneys can excrete in a given period of time.

What a Positive Test Means

BUN and creatinine levels both rise when kidney function fails; creatinine clearance falls. Normal BUN is usually 15 mg/dL, creatinine under 1.0 mg/dL, and creatinine clearance more than 80 ml/min.

What a Negative Test Means

Normal levels mean that kidney function is normal but do not mean that everything about the kidney is normal.

URINARY PROTEIN, PROTEINURIA, ALBUMINURIA

The kidneys normally do not excrete protein. These tests check for the presence of protein in the urine.

What a Positive Test Means

Kidneys that leak protein are abnormal. The more they leak the worse the injury. Normal levels of protein in the urine is under one-quarter gram in twenty-four hours. Over 4 grams a day is high.

What a Negative Test Means

Kidneys that do not leak protein are usually normal or near normal. Rarely, function can be abnormal even without protein in the urine.

PLATELETS

Platelets are a type of blood cell that helps in clotting. They are used up in severe clotting and are reduced by antibodies to platelets.

What a Positive Test Means

Low platelets occur for several reasons in lupus. All reasons need to be checked out, since very low platelets are associated with spontaneous bleeding. Normal platelet count is 150,000/cubic mL of blood.

What a Negative Test Means

A normal platelet count means no problems in this system.

There is a great need to standardize all lupus tests for use in laboratories across the country. Today, in some cases, one laboratory can show positive results for a test, while another may show negative results. Such confusion can interfere with the proper care of the patient and add to the emotional stresses that are abundant in the life of the lupus patient.

35

Kidney Biopsies

by Michael D. Lockshin, M.D., F.A.C.P.

About half of all lupus patients develop lupus kidney disease (nephritis or glomerulonephritis), so doctors treating lupus patients do several blood and urine tests to monitor the patient for kidney disease. Why, then, do doctors ask patients to submit to kidney biopsies? Don't they already know enough about the kidneys from blood and urine tests? What is a kidney biopsy, anyway? Aren't biopsies done mostly to test for cancer? Does a biopsy hurt? Is it dangerous? Is there another way to get the information?

These are some of the many questions my patients ask. Like most aspects of lupus, the answers often depend on the patient, but there are replies that are true for most people. I will try to answer some of the most frequently asked questions about kidney biopsies.

WHAT IS A KIDNEY BIOPSY?

A biopsy is a removal of a small piece of tissue for further examination. In lupus patients, kidney biopsies show the type and severity of inflammation and scarring. A doctor who asks a lupus patient to undergo a kidney biopsy is not looking for cancer. It is in *other* circumstances—not in lupus—that biopsies are done to hunt for cancer or deep-seated infection. The information a biopsy gives cannot be obtained in any other way.

HOW IS A KIDNEY BIOPSY DONE?

Before the biopsy is performed, a doctor does a urine culture to check for any signs of infection, since infection can complicate the procedure, and an x-ray (pyelogram, IVP) or sonogram to be sure that the patient has two kidneys and that both appear normal. Doctors will not perform a biopsy on a patient who has only one kidney or who has a malformed kidney. The biopsy procedure takes place in a hospital x-ray or sonography suite. The entire procedure takes an hour or two. The tissue removal takes only a few minutes.

About an hour before, the patient is given a tranquilizing medication, and an intravenous needle for blood transfusion is inserted in an arm vein (in case of an emergency). During the biopsy, the patient lies on her* stomach on a pillow to arch the back a little. The doctor, with a very tiny needle, numbs a small area of skin about halfway down the back and a couple of inches off to one side. The patient feels only a tiny pin prick. Then, looking at the kidney with the aid of an x-ray or sonogram, the doctor inserts the biopsy needle—it is about as thick as pencil lead—through the numbed area until it touches the kidney. At this point, he asks the patient to take a deep breath and hold it. While the patient holds her breath, the doctor quickly inserts the biopsy needle into the kidney and immediately pulls it out. The patient usually feels as if she has been punched in the back. She feels pressure, not pain. The doctor looks at the removed tissue under a low-power microscope to be certain that the specimen is satisfactory. If it is not, he may repeat the biopsy. He then sends the tissue specimen to the pathology laboratory. It takes a few days to get the final results back.

At this point, the patient returns to her room and stays in bed for several hours. Doctors and nurses check all the urine she passes to ensure that there is no blood in the urine (about 10 percent of biopsied patients pass blood). The doctor also checks the patient's blood count for a few hours to be sure that it does not fall. Presuming all goes well, the patient can then go home, often with no more pain medication than Tylenol. A dull ache will be present for a few days.

Sometimes it is necessary for doctors to do a surgical rather than a needle biopsy. This is more difficult than a needle biopsy. It involves surgical anesthesia, about a four-inch incision in the flank, and much more pain. If your doctor asks you to submit to a surgical biopsy, ask him to explain why a needle biopsy is wrong for you. There are some good reasons, but they are very individual, and fairly rare.

WHY DO A KIDNEY BIOPSY?

There is really only one answer to this question: to make a treatment decision. Blood and urine tests may suggest something is wrong with the kidney, but they do not tell the doctor enough. A biopsy helps the doctor determine how active one's kidney lupus is, how long any lesions have been present, and the amount and type of damage done to the kidney. Kidney disease causes no symptoms until it is very advanced, possibly too late to treat. It is best to treat before symptoms occur.

In general, a patient whose urine and blood tests (complement, blood urea nitrogen [BUN], and creatinine) are normal is unlikely to have serious kidney disease and does not need a biopsy. A patient whose kidneys are beginning to fail almost certainly has severe kidney disease; a biopsy in this patient will not tell a doctor something he does not already know. A patient who needs vigorous treatment for lupus symptoms that do not involve the kidney, say high fever or brain inflammation, does not need a biopsy, since she will be treated anyway. A patient who says she will refuse treatment for kidney disease (high dose prednisone and cyclophosphamide) does not need a biopsy, since the results will not make a difference in treatment.

The patients for whom a biopsy is most helpful are those who feel well, who are on little treatment, but whose blood or urine suggests kidney disease. Another type of patient for whom a biopsy can be helpful is the one who, after being stable for

---

*It is awkward to say he/she. For convenience, I'll say *he* for doctor and *she* for patient, and apologize to those who might be offended.

some time, shows an equivocal sign of worsening. Often the decision in this case is: is it worthwhile to treat this patient again? Also a biopsy is helpful if a patient has been vigorously treated but does not appear to have improved. The question is: Continue treatment, or back off and avoid treatment complications?

There are other reasons doctors recommend biopsies, but they are uncommon. The diagnosis of lupus, or at least of lupus kidney disease, may be uncertain. Sometimes the laboratory tests are confusing. A drug reaction may be the cause of the kidney problem. Another reason is research: to follow the effect of a new treatment. The doctor will explain if this is the case.

WHAT DOES A BIOPSY SHOW?

Doctors try to answer six questions when they do a kidney biopsy. The first is "Is the diagnosis of the kidney problems lupus, or is it something else, like a drug reaction?" Almost all of the time the answer is lupus.

The second question is "How active is the disease?" This is determined by determining the degree of inflammation of the kidney. If the biopsy shows a lot of lupus activity, the doctor will recommend treating it vigorously. If it shows a little activity, he will make a less vigorous recommendation.

The third question is "How chronic is it?" Chronicity can be measured by determining how scarred the kidney is. The higher the chronicity grade, the more the kidney is scarred, the less likelihood there is for recovery, so there is less reason to treat.

The fourth question is "How severe is it?" The meaning of the word severity is obvious. Lupus activity can be mild or severe or anything in between. So can lupus chronicity.

The fifth question is "How much is the kidney affected?" Focal disease means that it is limited in extent (patches here and there are inflamed). Diffuse disease means all of the kidney is involved. Diffuse disease is generally less serious than focal kidney disease.

Finally, doctors talk about "proliferative" and "membranous" disease. "Proliferative" (roughly) means inflamed. "Membranous" describes a type of thickening, or plugging up, without inflammation, of a part of the kidney called the basement membrane. When there is membranous disease, there is usually a lot of protein in the urine. Patients can have both proliferative and membranous disease at the same time, and many do. Doctors mostly want to know how much proliferative and how much membranous disease is present. They direct their treatment mostly to diffuse disease.

Patients will also hear doctors talk about light microscopy, immunofluorescence microscopy (IFM) and electron microscopy (EM). These terms describe the different techniques used to look at the biopsy specimen. Light microscopy shows inflammation best. IFM is best for showing abnormal antibodies that clog the kidney, and EM shows the basement membranes best. Most pathology laboratories do all three techniques on all biopsies.

The doctor's conclusion about the biopsy will take into account all these factors: activity, chronicity, severity, focal/diffuse, proliferative/membranous, as judged by light microscopy, by IFM, and by EM. With all these things to consider, it is pretty complex. Doctors often have to make judgment calls about an individual biopsy, so if the doctor hems and haws a bit in your case, it is because not all the features match perfectly. That is all right. Even in this case, the doctor knows a great deal more about you than he did before taking the biopsy.

IS A BIOPSY DANGEROUS?

Any time a doctor sticks a needle in your body, there is a risk that something will go wrong. The biggest risk is hemorrhage. Almost every patient has a small amount of internal bleeding after a biopsy. It is rare, perhaps one in one hundred biopsies, that the bleeding is severe enough to cause symptoms or to require a blood transfusion. A large amount of internal bleeding does cause pain and fever, and may delay discharge from the hospital. Blood that collects around the kidney after a biopsy can become infected. Very, very rarely a kidney is torn during biopsy and does not stop bleeding. In that case, the treatment is to operate and remove the kidney. In thirty years of taking care of lupus patients, I have never seen this happen after a needle biopsy. (I did see it happen once after a surgical biopsy.) Nonetheless, the minute risk of such a complication is the main reason why the doctor has to be certain a patient has two functioning kidneys before he considers doing a biopsy, and why doctors are not casual about any biopsy. An inexperienced doctor can miss the kidney and stick the needle in another organ. This should never happen. It is reason for a patient thinking about a kidney biopsy to ask the doctor how many biopsies he has done, and to be certain that an experienced kidney doctor is in charge.

Uncontrolled high blood pressure increases the risk of a biopsy. So does a bleeding disorder, usually low platelets. Drugs that affect the way platelets work, such as aspirin, also increase the risk. Allergy to the anesthetics or other medicines used during a biopsy is a reason not to do a biopsy. Kidney infection, a kidney stone, a blocked or otherwise abnormally shaped kidney, or a wasted away kidney are other reasons not to do a biopsy.

IS THERE ANOTHER WAY TO GET THE SAME INFORMATION?

In a word, no, but simpler tests allow the doctor to make a reasonable guess. A very carefully done urinalysis does give clues about inflammation. The urine has to be tested when it is very fresh, and has to be examined by someone very experienced. Most routine laboratories put urine specimens in a refrigerator and have a technician look at them late in the day, and thus they lose a lot of valuable information. Many nephrologists (kidney specialists) examine fresh urine specimens themselves in their offices. Blood tests and twenty-four-hour urine specimens can give an idea of the problem. For instance, it is rare for a patient with inflamed kidneys to have a normal serum complement. These tests are not very exact. A sonogram can show that kidneys are beyond salvage, but it cannot tell that kidneys are healthy. The bottom line is, sometimes, to make an intelligent decision about treatment, a doctor has to know what the kidney tissue looks like under a microscope, and that means doing a biopsy.

Don't be afraid to ask questions. Your doctor should be able to explain to you why he wants to do a biopsy, what he expects to see, and what he plans to do with the results. And you should agree that his plans sound wise.

PART SIX

The Doctor-Patient Relationship

36

The Doctor-Patient Relationship: An Introduction

by Henrietta Aladjem

"A *patient should ask their prospective physician if they have been a patient them-selves. Since I have had to cope with a prolonged illness, I give my love more freely to my patients, and now I need their love as well."*

—*Robert P. Shapiro, M.D.*

I have been fortunate to have had the finest physicians in this country take care of me. Some of them were: my next door neighbor Dr. Antoine Freed, a family physician; Dr. George W. Thorn, physician-in-chief at Peter Bent Brigham Hospital; Dr. Frank H. Gardner, chair of hematology at Peter Bent Brigham Hospital; Dr. Louis K. Diamond, pediatrician (though he treated me as a "grown up") and professor of pediatrics at Children's Medical Center in Boston; Dr. E. Donnall Thomas, a physician at Peter Bent Brigham Hospital, a Nobel Prize recipient, and an exceptionally kind man.

I recall Dr. Thomas walking into my hospital room carrying a tray with a huge syringe—a kind that I had never seen before. He saw my frightened look and said, "I am going to draw some bone marrow from your chest. It will hurt, but it is quick and bearable. I had the procedure done to myself, so I know how it feels." It hurt, as Dr. Thomas had predicted, but the fact that he was familiar with the pain made it more bearable. It hurt even more when he returned a few days later to draw more bone marrow from my hip.

Dr. Malcolm P. Rogers once said that the capacity of physicians lies both in their character and in the nature of their training. Dr. Rogers believes that medical students should be selected not only for their academic abilities, but for their interpersonal skills as well. He said that their teachers and the hospitals where they train should emphasize that medicine is an ethical, not commercial, enterprise. They will learn in large measure by imitating their teachers as models.

When patients ask me to what I attribute my long-lasting remission, I must admit that I really don't know. It could be the good medical care I have received at Brigham and Women's Hospital in Boston for the past thirty-eight years, or it could be strong genes. Or perhaps I am a living example of one of Canadian physician Sir William Osler's aphorisms, "If you want to live a long life, get a chronic disease and learn how to live with it." However, I suspect that the good doctor-patient relationship I had with Dr. Frank H. Gardner for several decades contributed to my emotional and physical survival. After my kidneys became seriously affected by my lupus, I was forced to acknowledge the effects that my disease could have on me, and with this realization came the frightening awareness that my condition could result in my own death. I forced myself to adjust to a day-to-day routine—one to which I was antagonistic at first and indifferent later. However, I gradually felt a widening sense of isolation engulfing me. I began to suffer from a sense of futility in my life. One day Dr. Gardner looked at me and said, "I know how you feel. I had tuberculosis shortly after I graduated from medical school. I had to spend many months in isolation and solitude." After his revelation, a new relationship evolved. My physician became a person who could help me, and I, the person who needed his help. Through our conversations, the doctor learned about how lupus affected my daily life, and I was learning about lupus, the disease.

He learned about the pains and dizziness I was experiencing, the fatigue and the malaise that were, at times, unbearable; he learned about my troubled fears of my becoming dependent upon others. He learned about my fears of losing hope, of apathy, of never developing my full potential, of giving up dreams, of death and dying, of leaving my three small children without a mother, and of my poor husband having to carry the burden all by himself. With all my problems facing the doctor squarely, it became easier for me to analyze my feelings and talk about those things. I could also discuss with him my home, the books I read, the music I liked to hear, and while the doctor struggled to help me keep my sense of self, he struggled to divert my thoughts from the illness and unnecessary fears.

Melissa Leung, a student at Wellesley College and a lupus patient once told me that "fear *bites*," and I have to agree with that.

Through those conversations, the doctor got a glimpse into my thought processes, and I became aware that he believed that the human spirit grew and developed even in adversity. I became more aware of his effort to touch that healthy part in me and direct it both towards helping myself and perhaps towards helping him to learn how to help me more effectively.

Perhaps it takes a physician who has experienced illness to understand a good doctor-patient relationship, or perhaps it takes a sentimentalist. Even though I don't believe that sentimentality is a virtue, I still believe that it is better than the heartlessness with which physicians treat patients today.

Dr. Frank Gardner is now Professor of Medicine at the University of Texas in Galveston, where he heads the Department of Immunology and Oncology. From time to time, I still talk with him over the telephone and even see him for a checkup. The last time I lectured in Houston, Dr. Gardner and Theo, his wife, came from Galveston so they could take me to stay at their house. Over the years, Mrs. Gardner and I have become friends, and when I stay with them, I feel as though I am with family. Dr. Gardner draws blood from my veins in their large old-fashioned kitchen, then rushes to his lab with the vials of blood. When he returns, I can tell by the twinkle in his eyes that all the tests were normal.

Sitting in their garden, the Gardners and I reminisced about some of the things we have experienced over the past forty years or more. I spoke about how short life can be and how grateful I was to have had those years to watch my children grow up and become self-sufficient and responsible for their own actions.

Dr. Gardner likes being a doctor, the way his father did before him. His sister, whom I met in Boston, is an anesthesiologist, and her husband is a general practitioner. Theo's father was the physician-in-chief at McLain Mental Hospital in Belmont, Massachusetts. This gives Theo lots of understanding about what it means to live with a busy physician.

What makes Dr. Gardner such a special physician? He has charisma . . . lots of charisma, and he is basically a caring decent person. It also helps that he has suffered through a serious illness. And it wasn't just he who had experienced illness—Theo had polio when she was young. She has completely recovered, but she, too, remembers what it means to be sick.

I remember when, during the cold winter days in Boston, Dr. Gardner was wearing a warm woolen scarf around his neck and a vest under his blazer. He took precautions against catching a cold. He never forgot that he had had tuberculosis . . . and he was careful not to allow it to recur. I, too, have to be careful not to rock the boat during my remission. As Dr. Gardner would say, "Don't change anything—don't experiment with new ventures."

During those short visits in Galveston, the Gardners and I don't talk about lupus. We are like friends. We talk about the fellows he has trained at Brigham, some of whom are now heads of hospitals, while others are important medical investigators. We talk about the Boston Pops and its orchestra's late conductor Arthur Fiedler. We talk about the Boston Symphony.

Sitting in the Gardners' garden, I recalled the night before I was to have major surgery in Boston. I called Dr. Gardner at his house. Theo, his wife, answered the telephone. She told me that Dr. Gardner was in the Midwest but she would find him and give him my message. The following morning, Dr. Gardner and my husband were both at my bedside before they rolled me into the operating room. After the operation, when I asked my doctor Dr. George Smith if the operation was successful, he answered, in his gruff but kind way, "Of course it was! That doctor of yours followed my scalpel as if he was doing the surgery himself."

Looking at the gardenia bushes in their garden, I recalled when Dr. Gardner was growing potted gardenias in their house in Belmont. Now their garden was full of gardenias, with huge blossoms of unimaginable beauty. In this setting, the blossoms looked like angels' faces under the blue sky and the golden sunlight. Dr. Gardner is very proud of his flowers. His sense of satisfaction is written all over his face. In my imagination, I could sense the affection expressed by the flowers, glowing a little deeper in their colors when Dr. Gardner was watering them.

One afternoon, Theo pointed to a huge egret perched on a log by the water's edge. She laughed when she said, "The bird seems to appear only when Frank is sitting here relaxing." I did not question her words, for I could vividly remember his huge black St. Bernard dog in Boston, who followed him around the house behaving like a puppy.

I always get carried away when I talk about my doctor. But forty years is a long time in a person's life . . . and all the Aladjems feel that Theo and Dr. Gardner are part of our family—part of our lives.

While my relationship with my doctor is extremely rare, a good doctor-patient relationship is important in the treatment of any illness. This section will examine the doctor-patient relationship.

37

The Partnership Between Doctor and Patient

by T. Stephen Balch, M.D., F.A.C.P.

The relationship between you and your doctor is an integral aspect of your health care. It must continually improve, so that you can benefit the most from it. It is not easy. Sometimes you may feel that cooperation is difficult and that you are at odds with your own doctor and have different interests. For example, you may want to hear more about your disease, while your doctor may have to hurry to see another patient. Or you do not want to take a medication because of its side effects, while your doctor recommends it because he or she wants your disease to improve.

IMPROVING THE PARTNERSHIP

The key to a good doctor-patient relationship is realizing that you and your doctor are on the same team. The effort must go both ways. The physician needs to be confident that the patient is capable of becoming an actively participating partner in the decision-making process. You, the patient, will have to accept some of the responsibility for the results of medical decisions and see to it that you carry them out properly.

In former times, doctors gave people very little information about their illnesses and expected blind obedience to their instructions. Today, we know that good compliance depends on a complete understanding of the instructions and the patient's agreement that the final treatment plan is a good one and can be accepted by both members of the partnership.

The partnership improves as you realize that you are the one in charge of your body. You know how it responds to different treatment and how it changes with illness. You are also the one to see that you treat it right; only you can see that the treatment is carried out correctly. Try not to assume that you cannot understand what is going on in your body. Patients also need to realize that the doctor is just as subject to the same moods, pressures, and errors that you are. There is no reason to be intimidated by your doctor, or to follow orders blindly.

Proper preparation is essential for establishing the kind of doctor-patient relationship that will allow the patient with lupus to be the best that he or she can be. As a patient, you must be prepared mentally, physically, and educationally for one of the most demanding roles in modern society. Following are several ways to help patients take full advantage of the doctor-patient relationship.

Full Disclosure

A good impression is certainly a great way to start. When you first meet your physician, come prepared to explain your health state and why you are seeking medical help. The more informed you are about your care, the more successful your treatment will be.

It is important for your doctor to know what you are feeling. Bring a legible list of your symptoms, the things that are bothering you, and the points you want to discuss with your doctor. Be as concise and precise as possible. Hand the list to the doctor if you want. This way, he or she can go over everything much more quickly without either of you worrying that you will forget something important.

During your first visit, tell your doctor about all the medications you're taking. You also need to mention any over-the-counter drugs you take; they could interfere with medication prescribed for you. If you keep a chart of your medication, bring it with you.

When seeing a patient for the first time, many physicians have no record of previous laboratory work or medical evaluations. They may waste a lot of time and money repeating tests that have been done before, perhaps recently. To avoid this situation, bring as many of your previous records of laboratory work or evaluations as you can. It is very important to remember that these test results may vary from time to time and from laboratory to laboratory. Attempts are currently being made to standardize many of the tests used with the lupus patient, and the laboratory your doctor uses should meet these standards. Also, bring a list of the names and addresses of your other doctors. And never assume that all the relevant information is in the records. Your memory and any record you may keep yourself are important sources of facts.

You can help the doctor gain useful information during the physical examination by understanding that he or she is looking for specifics. Doctors are not mind readers. They learn much from you by blood tests, physical examinations, and other procedures, but a large part of the information they rely on to diagnose and treat must come from you. Doctors try to understand what is going on in you from your symptoms. Therefore, they need your input and observations. Be as specific as possible about what you are feeling and thinking.

The Physician's Role

After your evaluation, your physician should discuss your treatment options with you. For some people, the recommended treatment may involve medications, skin care, alteration of daily activities, physical or occupational therapy sessions, or home exercises. (Therapy sessions and home exercises will differ greatly from patient to patient, so the physician and patient must discuss them individually.) The exact combination will determine your treatment plan. To arrive at it, your doctor needs to understand such factors as eating and work habits, exercise preferences, outside interests, etc.

Your doctor should also tell you the best ways to take your medications—for example, if you should take them with meals, or what might happen if you change your dosage on your own. Your doctor should explain the side effects that may occur. Some are potentially dangerous; however, most are merely annoyances. Often, physicians know ways of handling side effects that may occur.

Finally, it is often helpful to have your doctor explain to you how your medication works. For example, aspirin decreases pain and inflammation. The more informed you are about your care, the more successful your treatment will be.

After You Leave the Office

In addition to encounters with your physician, the doctor-patient relationship is continuous, even when the doctor is not present. You must help your doctor evaluate how well your treatment plan is working.

Keep track of your progress and follow his or her instructions closely. Record your responses for discussion at your next visit. In particular, pay attention to what factors make you feel worse or better, and note when you take your medications and how they seem to affect you. Consider if your treatment plan may need to be changed. This may be necessary if you are having trouble following directions; if you are having unpleasant side effects; if you cannot afford the medications; or if you are getting worse instead of better. Do not be afraid to ask your doctor to change your treatment; he or she will probably want to change something if you explain what is wrong.

If the medication becomes too expensive for you, look into ways to lower medication costs. One way is to ask your doctor about the possibility of prescribing generic (or nonbrand-name) drugs. These are often the same as brand-name drugs. You may also be able to get discounts on medications through an organization such as the American Association of Retired Persons. (They can be reached at 601 E. Street, N.W., Washington, DC 20049; (202) 434-2277.)

Working Together as Partners

There are other important areas of the doctor-patient relationship. Medical explanations are an area in which a perfect match between doctor and patient is difficult to achieve and describe. Each situation is unique. Different doctors handle medical discussions with their patients in different ways, and individual patients have different needs and expectations from their doctors.

Both the doctor and the patient should feel free to bring up the topic of referral for another opinion. Your partnership has little to lose and often much to gain by obtaining a second opinion, which will keep your diagnosis and treatment based on the best possible information. After you have seen the second doctor, you should talk to your regular physician and discuss any changes in your treatment plan based on this consultation.

The best way to describe a sound doctor-patient relationship is probably with the term "physician-directed self-management." This is a new name for an old concept that has been utilized in successful doctor-patient relationships for thousands of years. It follows the principle that the health care of all patients is only as good as the doctor's directions in managing it. In other words, the doctor is only as good as the patient's information, and the patient's success is only as good as the doctor's ability to work with the patient. Both doctor and patient should try to maintain communication in their relationship on a 50/50 level. If one or the other is not part of the relationship, it will not be successful. Patients should have a goal of having their doctors treat them the way they would treat themselves if they had the doctor's medical knowledge.

Physicians must set aside their image of themselves as the ones making crucial medical decisions alone, and instead undertake the less glamorous, more time-consuming process of exploring options and outcomes with the patient. Physicians often do not have specific training in participatory decision-making, and the methods of identifying a particular patient's preferences vary. Nonetheless, both the physician and the patient should make thoughtful efforts to spell out the values that affect their decisions. It is surprising to learn not only how revealing such dialogue is, but how effectively it creates a spirit of mutual trust. The team is complementary; you know a lot more about your body than the doctor does, and he or she knows more about medicine than you do. The key is to work together toward the goal of controlling a very difficult disease and improving your life as a result.

38

The Doctor-Patient Relationship in Psychiatry

by Malcolm P. Rogers, M.D.

There are special aspects of the doctor-patient relationship in psychiatric practice. For one thing, the examination of the mind depends upon the cooperation of the patient. Psychiatrists are unable to read minds. Each of us knows our own conscious mind better than anyone else does. We know our fears, our insecurities, our life experiences, our secrets, our feelings about others, and our views of the world as no one else could. We might not have thought it through or worked out conflicting feelings or shameful thoughts, but we alone possess the raw materials for such an exploration. So, from the outset, psychiatric treatment and evaluation requires a uniquely high level of cooperation and trust.

Becoming a patient generally requires a high level of trust. Patients need to trust that their therapist will maintain confidentiality and respect and be fundamentally committed to improving their well-being, as well as to doing them no harm. The latter means avoidance of exploitation, whether it be sexual, emotional, or financial.

THREATS TO THE RELATIONSHIP

These days, managed care excesses threaten the doctor-patient relationship. Sometimes it threatens the confidentiality and privacy of the relationship. Reviewers and case managers—often from distant 800 numbers—want the exact treatment plan spelled out at the beginning of treatment, and only then will they approve a small number of sessions, with further review required for further sessions. The reviewer, who may know nothing about lupus and relatively little about psychiatry, focuses on diagnosable mental disorders and standardized treatments. The subtlety of some of the dynamic issues of coping with a chronic medical condition and of sorting out possible organic from nonorganic causes may be lost on the reviewer. Furthermore, most managed care companies view all psychiatric providers as essentially equivalent. Special knowledge of or experience with lupus does not count for much. If the provider is not a member of a particular plan, then treatment with that person will in almost all cases not be reimbursed. The goal of the managed care system is generally to limit its number of providers so as to exert more control over the system. Their ultimate goal is profit, pure and simple.

BENEFITS OF THE RELATIONSHIP

The most explicit purpose in establishing a solid and trusting doctor-patient relationship between a lupus patient and a psychiatrist is to promote appropriate information gathering, treatment, and healing. In fact, the relationship serves multiple purposes: in allowing for the necessary flow of information, and, in itself, providing a vehicle for therapy.

The therapeutic aspects of the relationship bring many benefits for lupus patients. For example, there is often enormous relief simply from having someone finally understand what you are going through and how lupus affects you. When patients are seriously medically ill, there is so much focus on medical details that at times the human experience of the patient gets lost. For the patient, this exposure to hospitals and doctors may seem quite foreign and unrelated to most of his or her life.

Being able to describe their experiences and learn that others have experienced similar emotions or symptoms is very reassuring to patients. To not feel alone and isolated is to feel supported by a social network. Study after study has demonstrated the power of social support in buffering the adverse effects of stress and illness. Patients often find that support groups with other patients have the most potent effect in reducing isolation. Family, friends, and close doctor-patient relationships also have a powerfully supportive effect.

The relationship between a lupus patient and a psychiatrist may also be special in the freedom it allows for the discussion of sensitive or difficult issues, including the nature of the relationship itself, and relationships with the patient's other doctors, with friends, and with family. The psychiatric relationship may help to guide lupus patients in gaining maximum benefit from their other treatment relationships. Sensitive topics dealing with death, sexuality, and money are all quite appropriate within the psychiatric relationship and may be difficult to discuss with loved ones for a variety of reasons, particularly the desire to avoid burdening them.

Most patients with diagnosed lupus do consider the possibility of death, if only abstractly. Coming to terms with one's mortality and the threat of death is a frequent struggle for patients with lupus. Helping to instill a sense of hope and control is one of the most compelling benefits of a psychotherapeutic relationship. It may help patients to mobilize their own coping skills and resources, and to play a more active role in their own treatment. Helplessness and pessimism are among the worst manifestations of stress and depression.

When depression or anxiety has reached clinically significant levels, psychiatrists may not only prescribe medication to reverse these states, but may also help patients avoid self-defeating ways of viewing themselves or their problems. This can enhance a patient's sense of control and power. The expectation of improvement, which grows out of the doctor-patient relationship is generally referred to as the placebo response. It is a powerful effect, generally in the range of 30-percent likelihood of improvement. Until about 150 years ago, that was the only useful "medicine" that doctors could contribute. We have powerful drugs, but they can be relatively unhelpful when patients expect them to do more harm than good.

The doctor is also an educator about the disease and its treatments. The psychiatrist may have a particularly useful contribution to education. We are trained to start by listening and by understanding the patient's own ideas and theory about his or her illness. We have learned to ask a series of questions and to listen carefully to the answers. We might ask: "What do you think caused your problem? Why do you think it started when it did? What do you think your sickness does to you? How severe is your sickness? What kind of treatment do you think you should receive? What are the most important results you expect from this treatment? What are the chief problems that your sickness has caused you? and What do you fear most about your sickness?"

In every case, patients have answers to these questions, often detailed and explicit. They've been thinking about this much longer than the doctor. Effective efforts to provide information and care for the patient require such knowledge of their perceptions. They may relate the onset to some meaningful aspect of their lives.

39

Is *the* Patient-Physician Relationship Dead?

by Howard Steven Shapiro, M.D.

I *have known Dr. Shapiro for more than two decades and have admired him as a psychiatrist, a philosopher, and a good man. Over those years, he and I have often discussed the importance of a good patient-doctor relationship. His essay, entitled "Is the Patient-Physician Relationship Dead?" points out that physicians, when they become patients, have the same problems as we do.*

THE CHANGING FACE OF HEALTH CARE

Change is everywhere. All segments of society are affected and there seems no immunity from these upheavals. The very ground we stand upon seems to tremble, and we worry and wonder how to adjust and adapt.

What can patients do to help themselves to obtain adequate care when they seem to be caught between the ever-shifting sands of the medical delivery system and a public image of super-techno-cyborg medicine—the CT and MRI and PET scans, the lasers and the laparoscopes, the chemo-cocktails and the DNA codes?

Just who will qualify for all of these advances that make modern medicine so effective and expensive—so expensive, in fact, that the whole titanic health-care conglomerate is threatening to capsize? And, as we come to the surface, we see the writing on the wall—medical rationing ahead.

How did we get here? What can we do to cope . . . to survive? Before the advent of modern, "scientific" medicine, the patient-physician relationship was the principal means by which doctors could help patients mobilize and organize their own resourcefulness in order to get through a crisis. Doctors were the patients' and the community's gateway to the benefits and wonders of modern medical science. They were the heroic dispensers of miracles.

As the medical "industry" grew, the explosion of medical knowledge and technology shifted the focus of medical practice away from its *interpersonal* aspects and towards its *technical* aspects. Patients saw doctors as more and more "impersonal" but were grateful for the benefits of technical competence. An illusion grew: that anything was possible through science and technology, and past medical failures were due to human error.

The devitalization of the patient-physician relationship continued. Its disintegration was tolerated for as long as technical benefits were forthcoming. Its survival was barely nourished by those encounters at the bedside, in the office, or on the phone.

THE EFFECTS OF THE CHANGING FACE OF HEALTH CARE

"Progress" has turned out to be very expensive. The patient-physician relationship is in danger of strangulation by external economic constraints and considerations. Doctors' clinical decisions are increasingly aimed at high-volume, low-cost "efficient operation."

The so-called "crisis in health care" is forcing American doctors to relinquish much of their social authority and autonomy, and to work within a system of "health-care delivery" that is increasingly unsatisfying and unsatisfactory to both patients and doctors. Patients are "consumers," and health care is the "product." Doctors are workers employed by the providers, and patient care is replaced by cost containment.

Patients were once people with lives, families, and personhood; and doctors took care of their patients, who were well known to them. Doctors identified with their patients and felt their sufferings, fears, and hopes. Physicians felt their medical roots go deep and intertwine with the fundamental belief system of our entire culture. And doctors resonated with the identity of "healer," reliever of suffering, and health restorer. And this made doctors glad they had become doctors, whatever the sacrifices. Their patients knew this, and they benefited profoundly from the "human elements" in the patient-physician relationship that are either codified by or excluded from the new modular health-care delivery system.

Large business conglomerates want to survive and thrive. Their efforts to compete with each other and dominate their markets often sell the patient short because they disregard the aspects of patient care that do not fit as commodities. Those aspects of "health care" that do not fit their model of medical/economic efficiency often involve the human elements, and that includes in particular what is so specifically human, the patient-physician relationship.

SOLVING THE PROBLEM

The question is whether there are special or characteristic forms of communication and exchanges conducive to helping and healing and patient empowerment within the relationship of patient and physician. If there are, then we must make every effort to preserve or sustain those relationships. We must devise and implement a strategy to locate, identify, and obtain such care and to differentiate health-promoting medical care from "toxic" medical providers and systems.

In the first issue of *Lupus Letter,* Henrietta Aladjem emphasized that in addition to learning about lupus, she had to learn to "know her body, her spirit, and her soul," words that say so much about our humanness. Ms. Aladjem emphasized the therapeutic significance and importance of her close relationship with her physician. It was in the context of their relationship that communication fostered the development of understanding, trust, and respect.

The patient-physician relationship has been a subject of debate for as long as physicians and patients have existed. Our health-care crisis and the emphasis on patient empowerment has brought us back for another look at this age-old topic. Could it be that the physician can act as a catalyst or a template for a healing reaction in the patient? There has been much speculation about mind/body connection, healing, and the neuro-hormonal pathways that connect faith and belief to hard science.

What Can Physicians Do?

This year the *Journal of the American Medical Association* launched a new section called "The Patient-Physician Relationship." In an editorial, Dr. Glass states: "The patient-physician relationship is the center of medicine. As described in the patient-physician covenant, it should be a 'moral enterprise grounded in a covenant of trust.' This trust is threatened by the lack of empathy and compassion that often accompanies an uncritical reliance on technology and by pressing economic considerations. The integrity of the profession of medicine demands that physicians, individually and collectively, recognize the centrality of the patient-physician relationship and resist any compromises of the trust this relationship requires."

Doctors need to restore that trust between patient and physician and return empathy and compassion to "science and economics." Empathy is the most potent and important of all the therapeutic traits. Empathy is the ability to find out how someone else thinks and feels, and the willingness to understand their experience *as it is for them* without trying to interpret or modify it. Empathy also includes being able to connect with the person's feelings and responding to them. Obviously, it requires a degree of openness to one's own subjective states. Remember, empathy does not mandate the abandonment of objectivity, logic, reason, or modern scientific medicine. Doctors—good, wise doctors—use both objective and subjective thinking together. Dr. Jacob Needleman wrestles with this issue in his book *The Way of the Physician:*

> The doctor-patient relationship remains one of the last non-trivial forms of relationship possible for modern people. It must be kept within the fold of science because it is science, above all, that needs nourishing by the realities of conscious human energy . . . Don't let medicine become a humanistic discipline; don't let it become technology; don't let it become business. Keep all the science and with it keep the direct encounter between a human being in real need and another human being who is obliged to help him through knowledge of nature and attention to the human self in front of him."

What Can Patients Do?

If one is convinced that the patient-physician relationship is important, then one must be currently unattached and looking to hook up with a new physician, happily "married" to a current physician, or unhappily "married" to a current physician and contemplating finding a new one. And then there are all of those patients sucked up by managed care companies that deprive their "consumers" of choice by paternal-istically assigning them to various anonymous "medical providers" (whom we used to call "doctors").

If there is a choice left to the patient, what can he or she look for, in fact, strive for, in selecting a physician? And if choices are limited or impractical, what can be done to improve an existing relationship? Once you have made the decision and accepted the responsibility and the challenge to find "Dr. Right," you must then actively interview potential physicians rather than passively taking someone else's recommendation. Not unlike a blind date, it is only upon the actual encounter that you can sense if this physician is for you. You must be open to your inner emotions and feelings about the physician. Often that first impression or intuition is signifi-cant, especially when it is negative and warns that this physician is "not for you." Often a patient's fear, worry, depression, and hope for immediate help deafen him or her to his or her own inner better judgment in accepting a physician.

When patients have some choice, they should look for certain traits, which Jacquelyn Small calls "naturally therapeutic," in a prospective physician. These are empathy, genuineness, respect, warmth, immediacy, potency (competence), and a quality that leads one to sense that this physician desires to help the person, not just to treat a rash or disease. Typically this sort of physician is *naturally* a person who transmits his or her interest and desire to know the person who becomes his or her patient.

Ms. Aladjem spoke of the therapeutic influence of her physician, which led her to learn about her "spirit and soul" as well as her body. Patients should look for a physician who will confront them and who will challenge them to be more real, more truthful in their reporting, more self-observant, and more self-caring. In gen-eral, patients should look for physicians who:

- Seem genuine and allow patients to be themselves, not causing their patients to feel defensive or to role-play.

- Communicate by their very manner and interactions that their own inherent strengths and capacities are freely offered to their patients and that they accept their patients' considered choices, decisions, and mistakes.

- Do not fear occasional appropriate self-disclosures that are meaningful, perti-nent, and delivered with the clear intent of helping and comforting.

- Are not excessively judgmental or moralistic.

- Have that "human touch."

What can one do if locked into the care of a "Dr. Stoneface" or "Coldheart" and the prospects of a physician change are poor? One must recognize that with room for change, there is usually a way to make change. Empowerment implies the right, and in fact, requires the responsibility, to take action toward change, which may include confrontation.

I'm reminded of the time I had vascular surgery performed on my ankle by the most esteemed technical vascular surgeon in the area. A few days after the surgery, this doctor entered my room with not so much as a glance or greeting, bee-lined it directly to my ankle and mumbled to my ankle, "How's the wound today?" I quite spontaneously snapped back in a surprisingly loud but friendly tone, "Why, Dr. 'Stoneface,' that ankle you are addressing is attached to a leg, which is connected to a person, and that person is me. Perhaps you'd like to meet me someday? It can be arranged." The words stopped him in his tracks and, like someone finally "getting" a joke after an uncomfortable delay, he broke into a smile as he recognized that his characteristic bedside persona and behavior were my target. He missed the point of the comments, but the ice was broken. Some time later, he confided to me that no one had ever confronted him about his manner, but as a result of my actions, he had changed the *style* of his bedside behavior. (He still hadn't got it.)

This situation illustrates that with opportunity and effort you may influence the behavior of your physician. It also illustrates that one cannot change another's basic nature. What Dr. Stoneface could not change was his focus, which ideally should have been first, on the person he is treating and second, on the wound or condition of the person.

One should select a physician whose very nature includes being genuinely interested in people. This type of person should not be threatened by a patient's question, but rather should welcome and respect a patient's attempts to heal himself and willingly collaborate with the patient toward this end. Locating, developing, and enhancing the therapeutic physician-patient relationship not only insures the survival of patient empowerment but reinforces the kind of bond necessary to withstand the many socio-economic changes ahead.

40

Optimizing Patient-Doctor Relationships

by Peter H. Schur, M.D.

Few of us have pleasant memories of visits to a physician. Such encounters remind us that we have, or may have, an illness (a negative concept). We may then have difficulty dissociating that negative concept from the positive attitude we would like to have toward the physician, traditionally regarded as a healer. Why do we often consider disease as something "bad," rather than accepting it as something that is part of life, like paying taxes? Some consider even a short-term disease as punishment for something we did that we conceive of as "bad" or the result of an uncontrollable external cause.

Coping with a chronic illness such as lupus is so much harder to bear because the negative feelings about the disease linger on, as can the symptomatic pain and suffering directly associated with the disease. A chronic disease may result in physical scars or deformities; make housekeeping nearly impossible without help; create difficulty making meals, going shopping, dressing one's self, enjoying sex, having and taking care of children, and keeping a job; and result in a feeling of uncertainty and loss. Often, no external feature of the disease is visible, yet kidney disease, anemia, and psychological stresses may limit one's ability to adequately perform normal functions.

A sympathetic physician will try to help a patient cope with both physical symptoms and the feelings and perceptions about the disease. Unburdening one's self of fears and anxieties as symptoms are clarified often results in relief and reassurance as solutions are developed through effective patient/doctor dialogue.

UNDERSTANDING THE PATIENT-DOCTOR RELATIONSHIP

A relationship between a patient and physician is both a contract and a partnership. It is a contract in the sense that a patient contracts the services of a physician and agrees to pay (or have an insurance company pay) for the physician's service. The expected services are for the physician to ensure health and to treat disease. A partnership is important because it is imperative for everyone concerned with health to work on maintaining and improving it. That ongoing process means not only dealing with oneself but also working, sharing, and creating a program with a physician for maintaining and developing systems of dealing with disease when necessary.

Your good health depends somewhat on how well you relate to a physician. You deserve a physician's advice on how to stay healthy, when sick how to effectively treat the illness, and how to cope with the feelings you have about your disease. For that advice and treatment to be effective, one needs confidence in a physician based on a mutual sense of trust, which is a result of effective communication. Trust on the part of the patient, therefore, is based on having a physician who listens, explains, suggests ways of staying healthy, and treats you when you are ill. In turn, trust on the part of the physician is based upon a patient's practicing good health habits (including not smoking, eating well, exercising), being open and clear regarding symptoms and concerns, and following the physician's recommendations.

CHOOSING A PHYSICIAN

Different patients require different approaches from their physicians. Many simply want to be told what to do without any explanations; others want highly detailed explanations. Most fall somewhere in between. Most physicians will modify their style to suit a patient's individual needs; happily, most patients are flexible, too. However, sometimes it requires several different patient/doctor interviews to find individuals who can work well together.

In choosing a physician, one seeks someone who possesses superior knowledge about a particular disease; someone who asks pertinent questions and listens to the responses; someone who will provide answers and useful explanations; someone who is pragmatic and demonstrates determination to keep exploring avenues of resolution (especially important when dealing with a chronic illness); someone who is flexible and is willing to consult others when indicated; and someone who is cost conscious. But above all, one seeks someone who cares, offers hope, and inspires confidence and optimism.

A good family physician or internist is usually found through asking neighbors, friends, and family, and by contacting local medical societies, local hospitals, or a local medical school. Inquire as to why the particular physician was recommended—Is he or she board-certified (which indicates a degree of particular expertise). Inquire as to whether he or she is on the staff of a highly regarded hospital, and whether he or she is affiliated with a medical school (becoming a faculty member of a medical school is difficult and indicates that the physician is highly regarded by peers).

However, often a specialist is needed for a consultation for problems beyond those that even a capable and respected internist can handle. Specialists can be identified through the AMA directory of medical specialists, through the local medical society, or more easily through the local medical school. Your local Lupus Foundation may also provide such a list.

HOW A PATIENT CAN OPTIMIZE THE PATIENT-DOCTOR RELATIONSHIP

Arrive somewhat early for your office visit if forms have to be completed. If you expect to be late, call the office so that another patient can be rescheduled. If you need to cancel, call the office as soon as possible. Bring concise notes that list your symptoms. Bring copies of pertinent medical records, laboratory test results, and x-rays. Bring a list of medications you are taking, including their names (spelled correctly), their doses (how many milligrams are in each pill), and the frequency with which you take them. A list of previous medications taken, including whether or not they were effective and any side effects, is also useful. A discharge summary from any hospitalization is useful, as it is designed to condense relevant material into two pages.

Be prepared to describe your symptoms and how they affect you, the stresses in your life, your family history, your lifestyle (whether or not you smoke, drink alcohol, take any recreational drugs, exercise, or are following any type of diet) and your line of work. Bear in mind that your physician will have to spend some of the time allotted to you in scanning the material you've brought before a productive discussion can begin.

Bring along notes for yourself regarding what you want to discuss and what questions you need answered. Remember—there is no such thing as a dumb question. Be sure that before you leave, all your questions are answered. Remember that your physician has probably scheduled you for a certain amount of time for your visit. There is some time flexibility, but if your visit is extended, the doctor will be late for the next patient. If you can't cover everything in one visit, schedule another appointment during which you and your doctor can discuss your other concerns, and ask whether he or she has a specific "telephone time" for between-visit questions.

Ask your doctor what diagnosis or diagnoses are probable. Don't be afraid to ask for a layman's explanation of the illness or illnesses, and where you can obtain more information about them (physicians often have pamphlets available that describe different diseases). Ask about the seriousness and prognosis of these diagnoses and how they are best treated. Ask about alternative treatments and possible side effects of each treatment. Most medications are safe—otherwise they would not have been approved by the Food and Drug Administration (FDA). However, some side effects may occur, e.g., rashes, constipation or diarrhea, or drowsiness. Ask about the potential benefits and risks of medication. If answers are not clear, request clarifications. Take notes. Often a physician will write things down for you.

If you are in doubt about a diagnosis or specific treatment, feel free to obtain a second opinion. A capable physician will not be offended by this procedure, because he or she will be confident of corroboration.

Ask to schedule a follow-up appointment. Ask how to reach the physician in an emergency, as well as who covers on nights, weekends, and vacations.

Understanding Medications

No one likes to take medications, especially for a long time. Swallowing a pill is a reminder of the disease lurking beneath the surface suppressed by medication. The scenario is potentially psychologically demoralizing. However, when I prescribe, I do so because, based on my experience and that of my colleagues, the potential benefit far outweighs the potential risk. Discuss with your physician the goals for each medication: Is it pain relief, reducing inflammation, relieving anxiety, reducing side effects of other medications, restoring organ function, clearing up a rash, or enabling one to function? A positive attitude, i.e., focusing on the goals that medication will allow you to achieve, will help. Take medications as prescribed. Do not stop medications unless advised to do so. Stopping abruptly may cause a flare of lupus or a potentially harmful withdrawal reaction. However, if you have a bad reaction to a medicine, stop taking it and call your physician right away—if you can't reach him or her, go to a local emergency room for help.

UNDERSTANDING THE MEDICAL HISTORY

I encourage my medical students to read Agatha Christie mysteries as good examples of ways of learning to look, listen, and search for clues; for accurate diagnosis is similar to solving a mystery. Taking a history from a patient is a combination of reading previous medical summaries, listening (sensitively and perceptively), and asking pertinent questions, many of which may appear irrelevant, but certainly are not. Explaining the process of diagnosis often eliminates resistance to prolonged questioning.

My personal experience has always proven that no medical history is complete with just a list of symptoms. It must include a profile of the patient's personal life as well. A history begins with the patient's description of the symptoms and concerns that resulted in seeking help, and ends with anticipated goals ot treatment. Each sentence may evoke a question from the physician. A dialogue begins. Usually the patient begins with a description of symptoms. Ultimately, once the patient feels comfortable with the physician, psychosocial problems (such as problems with lifestyle, home and job situations, and juggling responsibilities of children and parents) enter the history as stressors, which may shed light on the underlying issues causing the patient's physical symptoms.

UNDERSTANDING TESTS

Signs and symptoms, no matter how eloquently described, are often insufficient to pinpoint a diagnosis. Doctors must, therefore, resort to and rely on modern technology and laboratory tests to acquire objective measurements that indicate what is occurring in the body. You see a doctor for lupus symptoms, and it seems to result in interminable tests. Some lupus doctors only test the patient and do not even take a history, listen to the patient, or even schedule an examination! Why the need for so much testing? Newly developed immunologic tests are so sensitive that they can now help distinguish lupus from other related conditions. In addition, these new tests for lupus often show abnormalities even before a patient develops symptoms. Tests also offer aid in distinguishing lupus symptoms (e.g., a fever, which may represent a lupus flare) from those that are caused by another disease. However, the sensitivity and specificity of these tests do not excuse physicians from meeting their responsibility of dealing with the "whole" patient, and how he or she responds to testing.

While occasional blood tests are easily tolerated, repeated ones can be debilitating. No one particularly cares to see his or her blood supply fill endless tubes and vials. As a physician, I am aware that the body manufactures new red blood cells each day. I can reassure my patients that anemia is unlikely to develop. Having to urinate often into a tiny bottle is messy and cumbersome. These are merely the physical discomforts. The emotional ones can be worse. Frequent testing is a reminder of the chronic nature of the disease. Fearing that the tests will reveal depressing news—especially when you are feeling better and thought you had just recovered from a relapse—can be very psychologically stressful. An anxious patient hears selectively what a doctor says and categorizes it in black and white terms—either good news or bad news. Tests with comforting results bring a sigh of relief, until the anxiety develops for the next round of tests, which may be days, weeks, or even months away. Disappointing results may mean even more tests, and perhaps more medication—with its potential side effects and its constant reminder of the problem.

Although x-rays are less painful than blood tests, legitimate concern about the dangers of radiation increases anxiety in patients. Fortunately, the newer machines tend to emit less radiation.

When all the aforementioned tests do not yield as much information as a physician requires to reach a diagnosis, a biopsy may be recommended. Organ tissue, when examined microscopically, will often reveal the characteristic tissue and cellular structure diagnostic of a specific disease. Some biopsies are relatively painless (such as punch biopsies of the skin, bone marrow, and pleura). Other biopsies can be somewhat hazardous (including liver and kidney biopsies) and are, therefore, usually only recommended when information anticipated from the biopsy far outweighs the risk of the procedure. Biopsies of more delicate organs, such as brain or heart, are done less frequently because of the potential hazard to the patient.

Other tests performed to assess various organ functions include blood counts (which assess bone marrow), urinalysis (which assesses kidney function), electrocardiogram (EKG, which tests heart function), electroencephalogram (EEG, which tests brain function), and blood tests and x-rays, which can be used to test the function of several organs. Which procedure will be used and the risks and benefits are issues that should be discussed in detail and at length by patient and physician.

Patients' rights include interpretation of test results. To help better understand technical details, physicians should provide literature that can help explain what the test results mean. Patients may ask for a copy of the test results (and/or other medical records); some physicians and hospitals will charge for this duplication service. These fees should be made known to the patient.

HOW PHYSICIANS CAN OPTIMIZE THE PATIENT-DOCTOR RELATIONSHIP

The patient's confidence in a physician erodes if his or her poor personal habits (he or she smokes in the office, is obese, or is sloppy) are evident. By extension, an office that is dirty, cluttered, and disorganized exacerbates the problem. On a personal level, patients are skeptical of a physician who does not examine them for a specific complaint, but instead orders tests and conducts a perfunctory examination. Physicians who are patronizing in attitude or terminology do no service to the relationship.

Dealing With Hospitalization

Hospitalization is often an area of confusion and conflict. Some patients actually want to be hospitalized, "to be taken care of," and think that definitive diagnosis can only be achieved in a hospital. They may feel, correctly, that insurance coverage is more comprehensive for hospitalizations than for office visits. But most people are unaware that admission often requires approval from an administrator. Many others are reluctant to be hospitalized and to accept how sick they actually are. They are afraid of dying alone and are unwilling to leave the security of home and family, fearing that their spouses and children cannot manage without them. All of these concerns are important and need to be addressed.

Dealing With Difficult Patients

An additional problem occurs when a patient requests unwarranted medication (such as antibiotics for a viral cold, narcotics, tranquilizers, or sleeping pills); refuses to diet, exercise, or stop smoking; and persists in demanding more and more detailed information (yet complaining that medical textbooks are too technical). A rare but related problem arises when a patient actually does know more about a subject than the physician. An honest physician will listen, accepting and appreciating the patient's insights. However, when the patient thinks he or she knows more about a particular subject than the physician, but really doesn't, dialogue is well nigh impossible and irreconcilable conflict can easily result.

Not the least of a physician's problems is a hypochondriac, someone for whom illness is a way of life. This type of person has a Ferris wheel of complaints and physician-hops, obsessed with the notion that all the tests and physicians have missed the "real" disease. These individuals are so preoccupied with their disease and their health that they may develop the illusion of controlling the uncontrollable with vitamins, jogging, dieting, etc. The chronic complainer loses credibility (the "cry wolf" phenomenon) as false alarms eventually fall on the deaf ears of family, friends, and physicians, who grow uneasy at the notion of missing a real illness. Difficult as it may be, the physician's role is to convince these individuals that an annual checkup usually suffices in pinpointing major diseases; and that an unresolved underlying emotional or psychological problem may be causing the "disease."

Physicians consider themselves both scientists and humanists. To correctly diagnose illness and treat it appropriately, physicians want and need to be objective. They need to be able to see, feel, hear, and measure something that can be defined as abnormal. Sometimes what a patient perceives as abnormal is not considered as such by a physician. If the imagined is all too real for the patient, that must also be dealt with accordingly. It is, therefore, important for a physician to believe the patient's reported symptoms. The art of medicine then can be blended with the science of medicine to determine the correct diagnosis and specific treatment, which includes how the patient can best deal with the problem. Kind words, sincerity, and a clear, comprehensible explanation of what is reality will help allay fantasies and fears. If a patient is having a great deal of difficulty dealing with his or her disease and/or its symptoms, consultations with a psychologist or psychiatrist and the use of specific medication may be indicated.

Dealing With Patients' Denial

Denial is a problem encountered by many physicians. Patients do not like to hear disquieting news, such as you do (or do not) have lupus, that you require a weight-management program, that you should cease smoking, that you should take (or not take) certain medications, that a conclusive diagnosis isn't possible yet, and more tests and/or consultations are recommended. A good physician is telling you what is in your best health interests. What can you do about the negative feelings you have about what is being said? Many patients simply go to another, even many other, physicians, until they find one who tells them what they want to hear. Assuming that one is dealing with a good physician, and most are, try dealing with your feelings about what is said, and do not dismiss the physician with the recommendations. Trust cements good patient/doctor relationships and in the long term will be beneficial in managing a chronic illness.

Both patient and physician should enjoy a mutual respect, set specific goals, and share responsibility for achieving those goals. To that end, the physician should instruct the patient on how to accurately monitor the course of the disease. Patient and physician should view the illness in a similar manner, and recognize that their relationship will alter as the other individuals (family members and/or consultants) become involved and as the nature of the illness itself changes, shifting priorities and requiring flexibility on everyone's part.

You want to be cared for by a physician; that is your legitimate right. You also have to accept responsibility for taking care of yourself as best you can. Together, you can make a great team!

Conclusion

What I Have Learned About Lupus as a Patient

by Henrietta Aladjem

I have learned about lupus from my own forty years of experience, from medical journals, from interviews with physicians, from conversations with patients over the telephone, and from the hundreds of letters I have received over the years.

I have found that it is not only the patients who find it hard to cope with lupus, it is also the physicians who are frustrated when they cannot cure the disease.

William Osler, the famous Canadian physician, once wrote that when he sees a patient with arthritis walk through his front door, he feels like walking out the back door. Since at that time there was little awareness of lupus, I suspect that the patients he was referring to were undiagnosed lupus patients.

Having been, for four years, a member of the National Allergy and Infectious Diseases Council at the National Institutes of Health has helped me to learn something about immunology and autoimmunity. I've become more aware of what is going on in my body and how to take better care of myself. I learned to stay out of the sun, eat a proper diet, stay away from harmful medications, and avoid stress as much as possible. I've also learned to budget my strength and to rest and exercise whenever possible.

Following is an excerpt of a conversation I had with Dr. Peter H. Schur, taken from *In Search of the Sun* (Scribner's Sons, 1988)

H.A.: Dr. Schur, I was diagnosed as having lupus in 1953. Do you think that lupus has changed in thirty years?

P.H.S.: Not really. Lupus hasn't changed, but our knowledge and understanding regarding it has changed considerably. Physicians have been better trained in medical schools and in postgraduate courses to recognize lupus in its early stages and treat it more effectively. Sensitive tests have been developed to aid in the diagnosis of lupus in its earlier and milder forms. Improved tests have also been developed to monitor patient therapy and fine-tune the doses of medications. A better understanding of the mechanisms whereby organs become injured and the development of many new medications and therapies have dramatically improved the prognosis for lupus patients.

H.A.: If the disease hasn't changed, have the physicians who treat it?

P.H.S.: Yes. Improved methods of treatment have helped physicians improve the outlook of the lupus patient from the medical point of view. However, physicians are busier than ever. They have more administrative obligations and must attend many hospital committee meetings. As a result, they often have less time to spend with a patient, and house calls are a thing of the past. Today it is unrealistic and logistically impossible to expect a physician to be all things to all patients!

H.A.: What do you personally consider to be potential problems in a patient-physician relationship?

P.H.S.: First and foremost, a patient needs a physician who inspires confidence and optimism. If there is uncertainty in either the diagnosis or the suggested therapy, a patient will tend to look elsewhere. If a physician is consistently unavailable, the process of disengagement will accelerate. The patient's confidence is eroded if a physician does not examine them for a specific complaint and, instead of ordering tests, conducts a perfunctory workup. Poor communication is another red flag. Physicians who do not listen, do not give adequate explanations, or are patronizing in attitude or terminology do no service to the relationship.

H.A.: What do you think characterizes the ideal physician?

P.H.S.: The perfect physician should be patient, supportive, and understanding of his patient's anxiety. He should have a solution for every problem, a treatment for every complaint. He is an excellent clinician, with a pleasant bedside manner, available day and night, and willing to give his home telephone number to his patients. Many older physicians fit this description well, having gained successful diagnostic and clinical experience over many years.

H.A.: What do you think characterizes the ideal patient?

P.H.S.: The ideal patient comes to the office with an accurate, concise, prioritized written list of symptoms, allocating a reasonable number of problems for each scheduled visit. Patients ideally should be cooperative, that is, be able to express their anxiety, anger, frustration, and depression, discuss their concerns regarding family, sex, friends, school, job, etc., and is willing to endure tests and procedures, is accepting of a period of uncertainty until a diagnosis is established, and is willing to suffer the often unpleasant side effects of medication.

H.A.: Assuming that neither physician nor patient fit these ideal descriptions, what do you think are the factors that contribute to a realistic patient-physician relationship?

P.H.S.: Both patient and physician should enjoy a mutual respect, set explicit goals, and share responsibility for achieving those goals. To that end, the physician should instruct the patient to monitor accurately the course of the disease. Patient and physician should view the illness in a similar vein, and recognize that their relationship will alter as other individuals (family members and/or consultants) become involved and as the nature of the illness itself changes, shifting priorities and requiring flexibility on everyone's part.

As I complete the last few lines of this book, I recall a young Canadian woman who died of lupus complications in a hospital in Boston. Her name was Ginette Proulx. In the last stages of her disease, Ginette insisted on coming to Boston to meet me in search of hope, or something to hold on to. I met Ginette at Logan Airport where she greeted me from a wheelchair. She was young and pretty, and her eyes glistened with fever and excitement. And I remember observing the girl, wondering where she found the strength to undertake this trip in her weakened condition? Was it her spirit that empowered her body to take such a strenuous trip? I wondered.

A few days after Ginette entered a hospital in Boston, she went into a coma. While her brother was leaning over her hospital bed telling her gently to hang in there because their mother was on her way to Boston, a nurse who entered the room said, "She can't hear you anymore." (Though I have read in several articles that those who are unconscious can not only hear what is being said, but can be disturbed by it as well.) At that moment, a tear ran down Ginette's cheek, asserting for the last time the power of her spirit.

Ginette fought vehemently for her life, but lost the battle. I've learned from this brave girl something about the power of the will to live, and I have also learned that one must assert life even at the edge of a precipice. I shall never forget that. I shall never forget Ginette Proulx.

Glossary

Acrocyanosis. Mottled blue discoloration of the skin of the extremities.

Analgesic. A drug that alleviates pain.

Anemia. A condition resulting from low red blood cell counts.

Antibodies. Special protein substances made by the body's white cells for defense against bacteria and other foreign substances.

Anticardiolipin antibody. An antiphospholipid antibody.

Anti-double-stranded DNA (Anti-DNA). Antibodies to DNA; seen in half of those with systemic lupus.

Antigen. Protein that stimulates formation of antibodies.

Anti-inflammatory. An agent that counteracts or suppresses inflammation.

Antimalarials. Drugs originally used to treat malaria that are helpful in the treatment of lupus.

Antinuclear antibodies (ANA). Blood proteins that react with the nuclei in cells.

Antiphospholipid antibodies. Antibodies to a constituent of cell membranes seen in one-third of those with SLE.

Anti-RNP. Antibody to ribonucleoprotein. Seen in SLE and mixed connective tissue disease.

Anti-Smith antibody (Anti-Sm). An antibody against a sugar protein found in those with lupus.

Anti-SSA (Ro antibody). A type of antinuclear antibody. It is associated with Sjögren's syndrome, sun sensitivity, neonatal lupus, and congenital heart block.

Anti-SSB (La antibody). A type of antinuclear antibody. It is almost always seen with anti-SSA. Also called the La antibody.

Arthritis. Inflammation in a joint with heat, swelling, pain, and redness.

Aseptic meningitis. Inflammation of the meninges (lining of the brain) that is not due to any (apparent) infectious agent.

Autoantibody. Antibody directed against the body's own tissue.

Autogenous vaccines. Vaccines made from the patient's own bacteria, as opposed to vaccines made from standard bacterial cultures.

Autoimmunity. A condition in which a person's body makes antibodies against some of its own cells.

B lymphocyte (B cell). A white blood cell that makes antibodies.

Biopsy. Sample of tissue taken for microscopic study.

Blood urea nitrogen (BUN). A product of protein metabolism. When the kidneys fail, the BUN levels rise, as do the levels of uric acid.

Bronchi. The tubes formed by the division of the windpipe, which convey air to the lung cells.

Bursa. A sac of synovial fluid between tendons, muscles, and bones that promotes easier movement.

Cartilage. A tough elastic connective tissue. The nose, outer ears, and trachea consist primarily of cartilage.

Chromosomes. Rod-shaped bodies in nucleus of cells containing the genes. Their number is constant in each species.

Collagen. Structural protein found in bone, cartilage, and skin.

Collagen disease. Group of diseases characterized by inflammation of the tissues of the musculoskeletal system. Usually synonymous with rheumatic disease.

Complement protein. Regulatory molecule of the immune response.

Complete blood count (CBC). A blood test that measures the amount of red blood cells, white blood cells, and platelets in the body.

Corticosteroid. A hormone produced by the cortex of the adrenal gland.

Cortisone. Potent hormone of the adrenal glands, also made synthetically.

Creatinine. A waste product of creatine metabolism. There are high levels of creatinine in the blood when the kidneys are not functioning properly.

Creatinine clearance. A twenty-four-hour urine collection that measures kidney function.

Cutaneous. Relating to the skin.

Cytokine. A group of chemicals that signal cells to perform certain actions.

Cytoplasm. Part of the cell that surrounds its nucleus.

Deoxyribonucleic acid (DNA). Basic constituent of genes. It is a large, complex molecule composed of sugars and nucleic acids.

Dermatomyositis. A chronic inflammatory disease of the skin and muscles.

Discoid lupus. Lupus confined to the skin.

Diuretic. A drug that helps to make more urine.

EKG (or ECG). Electrocardiogram, a recording of electrical forces from the heart.

Endocarditis. Inflammation of the inner lining of the heart.

Endocrinology. Study of the ductless hormonal glands and their related disorders.

Enzyme. Protein substance that catalyzes a biologic or chemical reaction.

Erythrocytes. Red blood cells, which have no nucleus and transport oxygen to the tissues.

Estrogen. Female hormone produced by the ovaries; it is responsible for secondary sexual characteristics in females and for the preparation of the uterus for implantation of the fertilized egg.

Exacerbation. Recurrence of symptoms; also called flare.

False-positive syphilis test. Some people, including lupus patients, can make antibodies to a fatlike substance structurally similar to the syphilis organism and consequently have a positive test for syphilis without having the disease.

Fibromyalgia. *See* Fibrositis.

Fibrositis. A pain syndrome characterized by fatigue, a sleep disorder, and tender points in the soft tissues.

Gastrointestinal series (GI series). An x-ray examination of the esophagus, stomach, and small intestine.

Gene. The biologic unit of heredity located on a particular chromosome.

Glomerulonephritis. Type of kidney inflammation characterized by involvement of the glomerulus of the kidney.

Hematocrit. A measurement of red blood cell levels. Low levels produce anemia.

Hematuria. Red blood cells in the urine.

Hemiparesis. Paralysis or weakness on one side of the body.

Hemoglobin. Oxygen-carrying protein of red blood cells.

Hemolytic anemia. Condition characterized by a reduction in circulating red blood cells due to increased destruction of the cells by the body.

Hepatitis. Inflammation of the liver.

Histocompatibility antigen (HLA). Molecules that can amplify or perpetuate certain immune and inflammatory responses.

Histology. The study of the microscopic structure of tissue.

Histopathology. The study of microscopic changes in diseased tissue.

Hormone. Chemical messengers that excite a response in other tissue.

Hypersensitivity. Form of allergy generally mediated by antibodies.

Idiopathic thrombocytopenic purpura (ITP). A condition of various causes, including SLE, characterized by very low platelet counts.

Immune complexes. Combination of antibodies with their corresponding antigens.

Immunofluorescence. Special technique of histology using a fluorescent dye to mark antibodies or immune processes taking place at a given site in the tissue.

Immunosuppressives. Medications that can suppress the immune system.

Interstitial pneumonitis. Atypical pneumonia due to either a virus or unknown factors.

Intravenous pyelogram (IVP). An x-ray examination of the kidneys.

LE cell test. The LE cell is a white blood cell that has swallowed the nucleus of another white blood cell. In the test, the latter appears as a blue-staining spot inside the first cell.

Leukopenia. Low white-cell count.

Livedo reticularis. Reddish blue netlike mottling of skin of extremities due to spasm of capillaries and/or small arteries.

Lupus anticoagulant. An antiphospholipid antibody that, contrary to its name, actually encourages clotting.

Lupus profundus. Inflammation of subcutaneous fat.

Lupus vulgaris. Tuberculosis of the skin.

Lymphocytes. White blood cells.

Lymphokine. Proteins made by monocytes and lymphocytes that affect other lymphocytes.

Lyse. To produce disintegration of cells, causing them to release their contents.

Macrophages. Cells that eat antigens, immune complexes, bacteria, and viruses.

Metabolism. Series of chemical processes in the living body by which life is maintained.

Mixed connective tissue disease. Consisting of two or more of the connective tissue diseases, for example, lupus, polymyositis, scleroderma.

Myasthenia gravis. Disease in which antibodies block nerve impulses from being properly transmitted to the muscle cells; as a result, muscles become weak.

Myocarditis. Inflammation of the heart.

Natural killer cell. Cell that kills other cells.

Nephritis. Inflammation of the kidney.

Neurosis. A disorder of the mental constitution arising from no apparent organic changes.

Neutrophil. Granulated white blood cell.

Nonsteroidal anti-inflammatory drugs (NSAIDs). A class of painkillers that work by interfering with the action of prostaglandin and by reducing inflammation.

Nucleoside. One of the four types of building blocks of DNA.

Nucleus. That part of a cell containing DNA.

Panniculitis. Inflammation of subcutaneous fat.

Pathogenic. Producing disease or undesirable symptoms.

Pathology. Branch of medicine that deals with changes in tissues or organs of the body caused by or causing disease.

Pericarditis. Inflammation of the pericardium.

Pericardium. A sac lining the heart.

Peripheral neuropathy. Malfunction of nerves of the arms and legs.

Peritonitis. Inflammation of the lining of the abdomen.

Pernicious anemia. Condition caused by vitamin B_{12} deficiency and characterized by anemia and spinal-cord abnormalities.

Phagocyte. Cell that ingests other cells or debris.

Phagocytosis. Ingestion by phagocytes of foreign or other particles or of cells harmful to the body.

Phlebitis. Inflammation of a vein.

Photosensitivity. Sensitivity to light energy.

Placebo. Inactive substance given to a patient either for its pleasing effect or as a control in experiments with an active drug.

Plasma. Fluid portion of the blood in which the blood cells float.

Plasmapheresis. Filtration of blood plasma through a machine to remove proteins that may aggravate lupus.

Platelet. A component of blood responsible for clotting.

Pleural effusion. Fluid in the sac lining the lung.

Pleurisy. Pain in the chest cavity.

Pleuritis. Irritation or inflammation of the lining of the lung.

Polymyositis. An autoimmune disease of the joints and muscles.

Progesterone. Female hormone produced during pregnancy that is primarily responsible for maintaining pregnancy and developing the mammary glands.

Prostaglandin. Any of a group of hormonelike compounds widely distributed in mammalian tissue that mediate a wide range of physiologic functions.

Proteinuria. Protein in the urine.

Psychosomatic. Relationship of the body to the mind; having bodily symptoms from mental rather than physical disorder.

Pulse steroids. Very high doses of corticosteroids given intravenously over one to three days to critically ill patients.

Purpura. Rupture of blood vessels with leakage of blood into the tissues.

Raynaud's phenomenon. Spasm of arteries to fingers and toes, causing them to turn white and later blue and/or red; may be accompanied by pain.

Remission. A period free from symptoms.

Renal. Pertaining to the kidneys.

Rheumatic disease. Any of many disorders affecting the immune or musculoskelatal systems.

Rheumatoid arthritis. Chronic inflammatory disease of the joints.

Rheumatoid factors. Antibodies to gamma globulin found in most patients with rheumatoid arthritis; may also be found in the serum of patients with any chronic inflammatory condition, including lupus.

Ribonucleic acid (RNA). A large, complex molecule composed of sugars and nucleic acid. It functions to translate DNA messages into making proteins, etc.

Scleroderma. A chronic connective tissue disease characterized by leathery thickening of the skin; the internal organs may also be involved.

Sedimentation rate (ESR). The rate at which red blood cells settle to the bottom of a test tube. Levels correlate with the degree of inflammation.

Serositis. Inflammation of lining tissue—usually either pleurisy, pericarditis, or peritonitis.

Serum. Blood from which cells and fibrin have been removed.

Sjögren's syndrome. Autoimmune disease characterized by dryness of the mouth, eyes, and skin.

Spontaneous remission. Marked improvement in a disease that occurs without medical intervention.

Steroids. Usually a shortened term for corticosteroids, which are anti-inflammatory hormones produced by the adrenal cortex or synthetically.

Subacute cutaneous lupus erythematosus. Lupus with characteristic skin lesions.

Synovitis. Inflammation of the tissues lining a joint.

Synovium. Tissue that lines the joint.

Systemic. Affecting the body as a whole.

T lymphocyte (T cell). Lymphocyte involved in cellular immunity.

Telangiectasia. Dilated capillaries and small arteries, frequently appearing on the faces of individuals with lupus, hypertension, trauma, and other conditions. They represent a scar, not an inflamed lesion.

Thrombocytopenia. Reduction of circulating platelets.

Thyroid gland. Gland located in the neck that produces various hormones, including thyroxine.

Titer. Highest dilution of a serum that gives a reaction with a substance.

Ultraviolet (UV) radiation. Radiation energy with wavelengths ranging from 200–290 nm (UVC); to 290–320 nm (UVB); to 320–400 nm (UVA).

Uremia. Marked kidney insufficiency in which wastes normally excreted by the kidneys remains in the bloodstream.

Vasculitis. Inflammation of the blood vessels.

Local Chapters of the Lupus Foundation of America

Alabama

LFA, Birmingham Chapter
4 Office Park Circle, Suite 302
Birmingham, AL 35223
(205) 870-0504

LFA, Montgomery Chapter
P.O. Box 11507
Montgomery, AL 36111
(334) 288-3032

Alaska

LFA, Alaska Chapter
P.O. Box 211336
Anchorage, AK 99521-1336
(907) 338-6332 (Phone/fax)

Arizona

LFA, Greater Arizona Chapter
2001 West Camelback Road, Ste. 135
Phoenix, AZ 85015-4908
(602) 242-2213
fax: (602) 249-2028

LFA, Southern Arizona Chapter
3113 E. First St., Suite C
Tucson, AZ 85716
(602) 327-9922

Arkansas

LFA, Arkansas Chapter
220 Mockingbird
Hot Springs, AR 71913

(800) 294-8878
(501) 525-9380

California

Bay Area L.E. Foundation
2635 N. First St., Suite 206
San Jose, CA 95134
(408) 954-8600
fax: (408) 954-8129

LFA, Southern California Chapter
17985 Sky Park Circle, Ste. J
Irvine, CA 92714
(714) 833-2121
fax: (714) 833-1183

Colorado

Lupus Foundation of Colorado
1420 Ogden Street
2nd Floor
Denver, CO 80218
(303) 832-2131 (Office)
fax: (303) 832-2114

Connecticut

LFA, Connecticut Chapter
45 S. Main St., Rm. 208
West Hartford, CT 06107-2402
(860) 521-9151
fax: (860) 523-9539

Delaware

LFA, Delaware Chapter

P.O. Box 6391
Wilmington, DE 19804
(302) 999-8686

Florida

LFA, Southeast Florida Chapter
6501 North Federal Highway
Suite 5
Boca Raton, FL 33487
(407) 241-5424
fax: (407) 241-6746

LFA, Northwest Florida Chapter
P.O. Box 17841
Pensacola, FL 32522-7841
(904) 444-7070

LFA, Tampa Area Chapter
Dibbs Plaza
4119-20A Gunn Highway
Tampa, FL 33624
(813) 960-3992

Lupus Foundation of Florida
4406 Urban Ct.
Orlando, FL 32810
(407) 295-8500

LFA, Northeast Florida Chapter
P.O. Box 10486
Jacksonville, FL 32247-0486
(904) 645-8398

LFA, Suncoast Chapter
P.O. Box 7485
Seminole, FL 34645
(813) 391-3000

Georgia

LFA, Columbus Chapter
233 12th St., Suite 819
Columbus, GA 31901
(706) 571-8950

LFA, Greater Atlanta Chapter
340 Interstate North Parkway, NW
Suite 455
Atlanta, GA 30339-2203
(770) 952-3891
fax: (770) 952-1760

Hawaii

Hawaii Lupus Foundation
1200 College Walk, Suite 114
Honolulu, HI 96817
(808) 538-1522
fax: (808) 521-8567

Idaho

LFA, Idaho Chapter
4696 Overland Road
Suite 512
Boise, ID 83705
(208) 343-4907

Illinois

LFA, Illinois Chapter
11102 S. Artesian
Chicago, IL 60655
(312) 779-3181
fax: (312) 445-8254

LFA, Danville Chapter
322 E. 13th St.
Danville, IL 61832
(217) 446-7672

Indiana

Lupus Foundation of Indiana
2701 E. Southport Road
Indianapolis, IN 46227
(317) 783-6033

LFA, Northeast Indiana Chapter
5401 Keystone Dr., Suite 202
Ft. Wayne, IN 46825
(219) 482-8205

LFA, Northwest Indiana Lupus
Chapter
3819 W. 40th Avenue
Gary, IN 46408
(219) 980-4826

Iowa

LFA, Iowa Chapter
P.O. Box 13174
Des Moines, IA 50310-0174
(319) 557-9324

Kansas

LFA, Kansas Chapter
P.O. Box 16094
Wichita, KS 67216
(316) 262-6180

Kentucky

Lupus Foundation of Kentuckiana
1850 Bluegrass Ave.
Louisville, KY 40215
(502) 366-9681

Louisiana

Louisiana Lupus Foundation
7732 Goodwood Blvd. #B
Baton Rouge, LA 70806
(504) 927-8052

LFA, Cenla Chapter
P.O. Box 12565
Alexandria, LA 71315-2565
(318) 473-0125

LFA, Northeast Louisiana Chapter
102 Susan Dr.
West Monroe, LA 71291
(318) 396-1333

LFA, Shreveport Chapter
2013 South Brookwood
Shreveport, LA 71118
(318) 686-2528

Maine

Lupus Group of Maine
P.O. Box 8168
Portland, ME 04104
(207) 878-8104 (Phone/fax)

Maryland

Maryland Lupus Foundation
7400 York Road, Third Floor
Baltimore, MD 21204
(410) 337-9000
fax: (410) 337-7406

Massachusetts

LFA, Massachusetts Chapter
425 Watertown St.
Newton, MA 02158
(617) 332-9014
fax: (617) 332-9685

Michigan

LFA, Michigan Lupus Foundation
26202 Harper Ave.
St. Clair Shores, MI 48081
(810) 775-8330

Minnesota

LFA, Minnesota Chapter
International Market Square
275 Market St. C17
Minneapolis, MN 55405
(612) 375-1131
fax: (612) 375-0102

Mississippi

LFA, Mississippi Chapter
P.O. Box 24292
Jackson, MS 39225-4292
(601) 366-5655
(800) 886-9606 (within Mississippi
only)

Missouri

LFA, Kansas City Chapter
10804 Fremont
Kansas City, MO 64134
(816) 765-3887

LFA, Ozarks Chapter
3150 W. Marty
Springfield, MO 65807
(417) 887-1560
(800) 328-8613

LFA, Missouri Chapter
8420 Delmar Blvd. #LL1
St. Louis, MO 63124
(314) 432-0008

Montana

LFA, Montana Chapter
29 1/2 Alderson
Billings, MT 59102
(406) 254-2082

Nebraska

LFA, Omaha Chapter
Community Health Plaza
7101 Newport Ave. #310
Omaha, NE 68152
(402) 572-3150

LFA, Western Nebraska Chapter
HCR 72 Box 58
Sutherland, NE 69165
(308) 764-2474

Nevada

LFA, Las Vegas Chapter
1555 E. Flamingo, Suite 439
Las Vegas, NV 89119
(702) 369-0474

LFA, Northern Nevada Chapter
1755 Vassar Street
Reno, NV 89502
(702) 323-2444

New Hampshire

New Hampshire Lupus Foundation,
Inc.
P.O. Box 444
Nashua, NH 03061-0444
(603) 424-5668

New Jersey

LFA, South Jersey Chapter
Starrett Bldg.
6 White Horse Pike #1-C
Haddon Heights, NJ 08035
(609) 546-8555
fax: (609) 547-6182

LFA, New Jersey Chapter
287 Market St.
P.O. Box 320
Elmwood Park, NJ 07407
(201) 791-7868
fax: (201) 794-8605

New Mexico

LFA, New Mexico Chapter
P.O. Box 35891

Albuquerque, NM 87176-5891
(505) 881-9081

New York

LFA, Bronx Chapter
P.O. Box 1117
Bronx, NY 10462
(718) 822-6542

LFA, Central New York Chapter
Maria Regina Center, Bldg. B
1118 Court St.
Syracuse, NY 13208
(315) 472-6011
fax: (315) 472-8634

LFA, Genesee Valley Chapter
P.O. Box 14068
Rochester, NY 14614
(716) 266-3340

LFA, Long Island/Queens Chapter
1602 Bellmore Ave.
N. Bellmore, NY 11710-5566
(516) 783-3370
fax: (516) 826-2058

LFA, Marguerite Curri Chapter
P.O. Box 853
Utica, NY 13503
(315) 736-5186

LFA, Northeastern NY Chapter
1533 Central Ave., Ste. 4
Albany, NY 12205
(518) 869-3856
fax: (518) 869-4368

LFA, Rockland/Orange County
Chapter
14 Kingston Dr.
Spring Valley, NY 10977
(914) 354-0372

LFA, Westchester Chapter
P.O. Box 8240
White Plains, NY 10602
(914) 948-1032

LFA, Western New York Chapter
3871 Harlem Road
Cheektowaga, NY 14215

(716) 835-7161
fax: (716) 835-7251

LFA, New York Southern Tier
Chapter
19 Chenango St., Suite 410
Binghamton, NY 13901
(607) 772-6522

SLE Foundation
149 Madison Ave.
New York, NY 10016
(212) 685-4118
fax: (212) 545-1843

North Carolina

LFA, Charlotte Chapter
101 Colville Road
Charlotte, NC 28207
(704) 375-8787

LFA, Raleigh Chapter
P.O. Box 10171
Raleigh, NC 27605
(919) 772-8564

LFA, Winston-Triad Lupus Chapter
NCLF
2841 Foxwood Lane
Winston Salem, NC 27103
(910) 768-1493 (Phone/fax)

Ohio

LFA, Akron Area Chapter
942 N. Main St. #23
Akron, OH 44310
(216) 253-1717

LFA, Columbus, Marcy Zitron
Chapter
6161 Busch Blvd., Ste. 76
Columbus, OH 43229
(614) 846-9249 (Office)

LFA, Greater Cleveland Chapter
20524 1/2 Southgate Park
Maple Heights, OH 44137
(216) 531-6563

LFA, Northwest Ohio Lupus Chapter
1615 Washington Ave.

Findlay, OH 45840
(419) 423-9313

Oklahoma

Oklahoma Lupus Association
3131 N. MacArthur, Suite 140D
Oklahoma City, OK 73122
(405) 495-8787

Pennsylvania

LFA, Delaware Valley Chapter
44 W. Lancaster Ave.
Ardmore, PA 19003
(610) 649-9202
fax: (610) 649-7549

LFA, Northeast Pennsylvania Chapter
c/o James/Alice Klas
822 Ash Ave.
Scranton, PA 18510
(717) 342-6146

LFA, Northwestern Pennsylvania
Chapter
P.O. Box 885
Erie, PA 16512-0885
(814) 866-0226

LFA, Western Pennsylvania Chapter
1323 Forbes Ave., Suite 200
Pittsburgh, PA 15219
(412) 261-5886
fax: (412) 471-2722

Lupus Foundation of Philadelphia
Thomas Jefferson University
Ford Road Campus
3905 Ford Road, 2nd Floor
Philadelphia, PA 19131
(215) 578-3515

Rhode Island

LFA, Rhode Island Chapter
#8 Fallon Ave.
Providence, RI 02908
(401) 421-7227

South Carolina

LFA, South Carolina Chapter
P.O. Box 7511

Columbia, SC 29202
(803) 794-1000
fax: (803) 794-7721

For UPS:
LFA, South Carolina
1038 Center Street
West Columbia, SC 29169

Tennessee

LFA, East Tennessee Chapter
5612 Kingston Pike, Suite 5
Knoxville, TN 37919
(423) 584-5215

LFA, Memphis Area Chapter
3181 Poplar Ave., Suite 100
Memphis, TN 38111
(901) 458-5302 (Office)

LFA, Nashville Area Chapter
2200 21st Ave., Suite 253
Nashville, TN 37212-4929
(615) 298-2273

Texas

El Paso Lupus Association
P.O. Box 4965
El Paso, TX 79914-4965
(915) 751-6941

LFA, North Texas Chapter
14465 Webb Chapel, Ste. 206
Dallas, TX 75234
(214) 484-0503
fax: (214) 484-0991

LFA, Texas Gulf Coast Chapter
3100 Timmons Lane #410
Houston, TX 77027
(713) 623-8267
fax: (713) 965-9051

LFA, South Central Texas Chapter
McCullough Medical Center
4118 McCullough Ave. #19
San Antonio, TX 78212-1968
(210) 824-1344
fax: (210) 824-3028

LFA, West Texas Chapter

1717 Avenue K, Suite 127
Lubbock, TX 79401
(806) 744-6666

Utah

LFA, Utah Chapter, Inc.
45 East Gentile
Layton, UT 84041
(801) 593-0921

Vermont

LFA, Vermont Chapter
P.O. Box 115
Waterbury, VT 05676
(802) 244-5988

Virginia

LFA, Central Virginia Chapter
P.O. Box 25418
Richmond, VA 23260-5418
(804) 270-1626 (Office)

LFA, Eastern Virginia Chapter
Pembroke One
281 Independence Blvd., Ste. 442
Virginia Beach, VA 23462
(804) 490-2793

Washington DC

Lupus Foundation of Greater
Washington
515 A Braddock Road, 2C
Alexandria, VA 22314
(703) 684-2925
fax: (703) 684-2927

West Virginia

LFA, Kanawha Valley Chapter
P.O. Box 8274
South Charleston, WV 25303
(304) 529-2600

Wisconsin

The Lupus Society of Wisconsin
1568 S. 24th St.
Milwaukee, WI 53204-2505
(414) 643-8522

INTERNATIONAL ASSOCIATED GROUPS

Argentina

ALUA (Asociación Lupus Argentina)
Angeles Pareja-Sackmann
Aguero 2345 5 "E"
1425 Buenos Aires
Argentina

Australia

Arthritis Foundation of Queensland
P.O. Box 901
Toowong, Queensland 4066
Australia

Lupus Support Group Queensland
42 Jainba Street
Indooroopilly, Queensland 4068
Australia

Lupus Association of Tasmania, Inc.
Box 404
Rosny Park
Tasmania, 7018
Australia

Lupus/Scleroderma Group
Arthritis Foundation of Australia, SA
99 Anzac Highway
Ashford, S. Australia 5035
Australia
Phone: (08) 297-2488

Victorian Lupus Association
attn: Enid Elton
Box 811 F, G.P.O.
Melbourne, Victoria 3001
Australia
Phone: (03) 650-5348

Lupus Association of NSW, Inc.
P.O. Box 89
North Ryde, NSW 2113
Australia
Lupus Group of WA (Inc.)
P.O. Box U1956
Perth, Western Australia 6845
Australia

Riverina Lupus Support Group
5 Pearson St.
Uranquinty, NSW 2652
Australia

Belgium

Liga Voor Chronische Inflammatoire
Bindweefselziekten
Ganzendries 34
B-9420 Erpe-Mere
Belgium

Bermuda

The Lupus Association of Bermuda
P.O. Box HM 1291
Hamilton HM FX
Bermuda

Brazil

Cristiano A.F. Zerbini, MD
Lupus Society of Brazil
Rua Padre Garcia Velho 72
Sao Paulo, SP 05421
Brazil

Maria da Conceicao Lopes Buarqu
Joice Romanini
Cx. Postal 68009
CEP 21944 - Cidade Universitaria
Ilha do Fundao
Rio de Janeiro, Brasil

Bulgaria

LFA Chapter Phillipopolis
attn: Dr. Emilie Spassova
2 Yosif Shniter Street
4000 Plovdiv
Bulgaria

Canadian Provinces

Alberta

Lupus Society of Alberta
North Tower, Rm 262, Foothills
Hospital
1403 29 Street NW
Calgary, Alberta T2N 2T9
Canada

Lupus Canada
(address same as LE Society of
Alberta)

British Columbia
British Columbia Lupus Society
Ross Pattee
433 E. 2nd Street
North Vancouver, BC V7L 1C9
Canada

(Residence)
Valley Lupus Group
attn: Ms. Robin C. Hay
34160 Palace Court
Abbotsford, BC V2S 6P7
Canada

Manitoba
Arthritis Self Help Group
attn: Ruth Kuch
825 Sherbrook Street
Winnipeg, Manitoba R3A 1M5
Canada

Lupus Society of Manitoba
attn: Mabel Wood, Pres.
RR #3
Carman, Manitoba R0G 0J0
Canada

New Brunswick
Lupus New Brunswick
attn: Ms. Lavina Townes, Pres.
Box 429
McAdam, New Brunswick E0H 1K0
Canada

Newfoundland
Lupus Society of Newfoundland
Box 8824
Manuels, Newfoundland A1X 1C4
Canada

Nova Scotia
Lupus Society of Nova Scotia
attn: Mrs. Lynda Cavanagh, Pres.
71 Penhorn Dr.
Dartmouth, Nova Scotia B2W 1K8
Canada

Ontario
The Ontario Lupus Association
attn: Stewart Stainton, Pres.
250 Bloor St. E Suite 901
Toronto, Ontario M4W 3P2
Canada

The Lupus Society of Hamilton
Jackson Station
Box 57414
Hamilton, Ontario L8P 4X2
Canada

Lupus Foundation of Ontario
attn: Mrs. Rhoda Mangus
Box 687
Ridgeway, Ontario L0S 1N0
Canada

Quebec
Lupus Québec
24 ouest, du Mont Royal, C.P. #8:
Suite 602
Montréal, Québec H2T 2S2
Canada

Prince Edward Island
Affiliated Support Group
Lupus Society of P.E.I.
Box 23002
Charlottestown, P.E.I. C1E 1Z6

Saskatchewan
The Lupus Erythematosus Society of
Saskatchewan
attn: Betty Bellamy
Box 88, Royal University Hospital
Saskatoon, Saskatchewan S7N 0W0
Canada

L.E.S.S. Prince Albert Chapter
P.O. Box 473
Prince Albert, Saskatchewan S6V 5R8
Canada

L.E.S.S. Regina Chapter
attn: Janet Erickson, Pres.
P.O. Box 3881
Regina, Saskatchewan S4P 3R8
Canada

Chile

Chilean Lupus Foundation
Iris Rivas P., Presidente
Avda. Bulnes 180 Dp. 50
Santiago
Chile

China

Zhang Xin, Chief - Dept. of
Rheumatology
Xian Fifth Hospital
Xian City
Rhaanxi Province 710082
Peoples Republic of China

Colombia

Diana Delgado H.
K 14 N 142-95
Bogotá
Colombia

Czechoslovakia

Professor Karel Trnavsky, MD, DSC
President, Institute of Rheumatology
Na slupi 4 128 50
Praha 2, Czechoslovakia

Ecuador

Fundación Lupus Eritematoso
attn: Rosario H. Solorzano de Gumsly
Casilla Postal 99-C Sucursal 15
Quito
Ecuador

England

Rookery Nook
attn: Cheryl N. Marcus
17 Monkhams Dr.
Woodford Green, Essex IG8 0LG
England

Lupus UK
P.O. Box 999
Romford, Essex RM1 1DW
England

United Kingdom Lupus Group
Arthritis Care

18 Stephenson Way
London NW1 2HD
England

Luton District Lupus Group
19 High Mead
Luton, Bedsford LU3 1RY
England

Liverpool Lupus Group
53 Westbourne Ave.
Thornton, Liverpool L23 10P
England

France

Association Francaise des Lupiques
attn: Mde. Andrés Harnon, Pres.
25 rue des Charmettes
69100 Villeurbanne
France

AFL European Intercontinental
Commission
165 Bd. de Stalingrad
69006 Lyon
France

Germany

Lupus Erythematodes
Selbsthilfegemeinschaft e.v.
Karin Hilmer
Gollemkamp 3
4600 Dortmund 15
Germany

Rheuma-Ambulanz
attn: Dr. E. Schmidt-Hengst
Medizinische Universitats-Poliklinik
Wilhelmstr, 35-37
5300 Bonn 1
Germany

Deutsche Rheuma-Liga
Landesverband Hessen e.v.
Birgitt Klatt
L.E. Arbeitskreis
Eulengasse 3
6000 Frankfurt am Main 60
Germany

Holland

Peter C.W.A. Bakker
Nationele Vereniging
L.E. Patienten
Bisonspoor 3004
3605 LV Maarssen
Holland

Lupus Patienten Groep
Juul Gerritsen
Thorbeckesingel 106
7204 KV Zutphen
Holland

Ireland

Lupus Support Group, Ltd.
Mrs. Catherine Delaney
40 Killester Park
Dublin 5
Ireland

Cork Branch
Mrs. Maire de Baroid
3 Ard na Greine
Evergreen Road, Cork 4 Ireland

Israel

Israel Lupus Association
attn: Mrs. Margalit Nusinov
P.O. Box 473
Ra'anana
Israel

Italy

Prof. Albert Marmont
Direttore Divisione de Ematologica E
di Immunologica Clinica
Ospedale S. Martino XIII U.S. L.
Viale Benedetto XV, 10
16132 Genova
Italy

Vena Gino Antoniao, Associate
Professor
Clinica Dermatologica Universita
Policlinico P. za Giulio Cesare
70100 Bari

Japan

Susumu Sugai, MD
Kanazawa Medical University
Uchinada - Machi, Kahokugun
Ishikawa - Ken 920-02
Japan

Malaysia

Malaysian Society of Rheumatology
Dr. Gek Liew Chin
26 Persiaran Jelutong
Damansara Heights
50490 Kuala Lumpur
Malaysia

Mexico

Dr. J. Humberto Orozco-Medina
Club de Lupus Centro Médico del
Occidente
Pedro Buzeta 870-B
44660 Guadalajara, Jalisco
México

Morocco

Assoc. of Lupus Victims of Morocco
Akhlij Fatna
40 rue des Alpes Maarif
Casablanca Morocco

New Zealand

Lupus Association of New Zealand
c/o Arthritis Rheumatism Foundation
of New Zealand, Inc.
P.O. Box 10-020
Wellington
New Zealand

Nigeria

Lupus Awareness Association of
Nigeria
attn: Agu Emmanuel Elochukwu
P.O. Box 30, Owelli
Awgu Local Government Area
Enugu State, Nigeria

Panama

Fundación de Lupus de Panama
Ana Elvira Brewer, Pres.
P.O. Box 7877
Panama 9
Republic of Panama

Paraguay

Vivan Ayala
Casill de Correo 2031
Asunción
Paraguay

Philippines

Arthritis Foundation of the
Philippines, Inc.
Tito P. Torralba, MD, Chairman
c/o Santo Tomas University Hospital
Room 216-B
España Street
Manila
Philippines

Analiza A. Panucial
Sr. Osmena St.
Lapu-Lapu City 6015
Philippines

Poland

Instytut Reumatologiczny
attn: Dr. Henryka Maldykowa
ul. Spartanska 1
02-637 Warszawa
Poland

Portugal

Prof. Viana de Queiroz
Universidade de Lisboa
Hospital Universitario de Santa Maria
Av. Prof Egas Moniz
1699 Lisboa
Portugal

Puerto Rico

Apoyo-L
Michael Ortiz
Del Carmen #7
Juana Diaz, PR 00795

Romania

Clinica Dermatologica Cluj-Napoca
Dr. Nicolae Maier, Chief
str. Clinicilor nr. 3
3400 Cluj-Napoca
Romania

Scotland

Strathclyde Lupus Group
attn: Mrs. Jane Elliott
6 Hawkhead Road
Paisley PA1 3NA
Scotland

Singapore

Dr. Feng Pao Hsii, Vice-Chairman
National Arthritis Fndn. of Singapore
336 Smith St. #06-302
New Bridge Center 0105
Singapore

South Africa

Lupus Support Group
Yvonne Bowker
Box 653
Somerset West 7129
South Africa

Lupus Support of Johannesburg
Mrs. Helena Hurwitz
P.O. Box 85316, Emmarentia 2029
Johannesburg
South Africa

Spain

Spanish SLE Aid Group
Dr. Josep Font
Hospital Clinic, Dept. Internal
Medicine, Unit 1
Villarroel 170
08036 Barcelona
Spain

Fundación Jimenez Díaz
Dr. Rafael Munoz Blanch
Clínica de Ntra. Sra. de la
Concepción
Avda. Reyes Católicos No. 2

Madrid (Ciudad Universitaria) 28040
Spain

Miguel A. de Frutos-Sanz
La Espuela, 26
29016 Málaga
Spain

Catalunya Association of L.E.
attn: Montserrat Pérez, MD
Hosp. Santa Creu i Sant Pau -
Barcelona

Dept. Dermatología
Avda. Sant A.M. Claret 167
08025 Barcelona
Spain

Asociación de Lúpicos de Andalucia
c/Martinez de La Rosa
No. 155-157, 1-B, Esc. Drcha.
29010 Málaga
Spain

Grupo Lupus de Madrid
attn: Elean Trueba
c/ Alvstante, 3
28002 Madrid
Spain

Sweden

SLE-Gruppen i RMR
P.O. Box 12851

S-112 98 Stockholm
Sweden

Switzerland

Selbsthilfegruppe for SLE
c/o Gabriela Quenson
Wellhauserweg 42
8500 Frauenfeld
Switzerland

West Indies

Lupus Society of Trinidad Tobago
attn: Curtis Wilson, Pres.
c/o Skin Clinic, General Hospital
Charlotte Street
Port of Spain, Trinidad
West Indies

The Hope Foundation of Barbados
attn: Shelley Weir
112 First Avenue, Pelican
Husband Gardens
St. James, Barbados
West Indies

Lupus Foundation of Jamaica
The Resource Center
attn: Mrs. Blossom Watson
1 Meadowbrook Main
Kingston 19, Jamaica
West Indies

Index

Positron emission tomography (PET),
    108
Prednisone. *See* Steroids.
Pregnancy, 67, 74
    antiphospholipid antibody and,
        71-72, 155
    delivery, 72
    flares during, 67-69
    kidney disease and, 69
    medication, use of, during, 69, 154
    monitoring lupus during, 69-70,
        153-154
    renal disease and, 155
    risks of, 70-71
    thrombocytopenia and, 155
    treating symptoms during, 153-154
    See also Neonatal lupus.
Prolactin, 65
Psychiatric manifestations
    medication for, 165-169
    resulting from medication, 163-165
    treatment of, 151-152
    types of, 103-106
    See also Neuropsychiatric
    manifestations.
Psychiatry, 32, 33
    doctor-patient relationship in,
        195-197
Psychic energizers, 168-169
Psychological effects of lupus. *See*
    Lupus, psychological effects of
    having.
Psychological testing, 107
Psychology, 32, 33
Psychosis, 10, 103-104

Radionuclide brain scanning, 108
Rashes. *See* Skin rashes.
Raynaud's phenomenon, 38-39, 159
Red blood cells, 113
Rodnan, Gerald, 37-40
Rothfield, Naomi, 29

Salicylates, side effects of, 163
Schur, Peter H., 40, 89, 213-214
Seizures, 9, 100-101
Self-efficacy, 45

Senne, Peter, 23-24
Silver, Robert, 31-35
Single photon emission computed
    tomography (SPECT) scanning,
    108
Skeletal complications, 83-84
Skin rashes, 115-116
    diagnosis of, 118-119
    therapy for, 119
    types of, 116-118
    See also Epidermal lesions;
    Photosensitivity.
Social science, 32, 33
Spectroscopy, 108
Steroids, 132-135
    side effects of, 165
Stress, managing, 45-46
Stroke, 100
Systemic lupus erythematosus (SLE).
    See Lupus.

Telogen effluvium, 118
Tests
    types of, 106-107, 173-178
    understanding, 208-209
Thrombocytopenia, 113-114
    pregnancy and, 155
    treatment of, 149-150
Thrombophlebitis. *See* Venous
    thrombosis.
Thrombosis, 118. *See also* Venous
    thrombosis.
T-lymphocytes, 122

Ultraviolet light, 121-122

Vasculitis, 118
Venous thrombosis, 94
Verrucae, 91

Warts. *See* Verrucae.
White blood cell injections, 130
White blood cells, 114
Women, lupus in, 57-58. *See also*
    Menopause.
Workplace, lupus and. *See* Lupus,
    workplace adjustments and.